MW00583175

PALEO SALADS

100+ ORIGINAL PALEO SALAD RECIPES FOR MASSIVE WEIGHT LOSS AND A HEALTHY LIFESTYLE

By Elena Garcia

Holistic Wellness Books

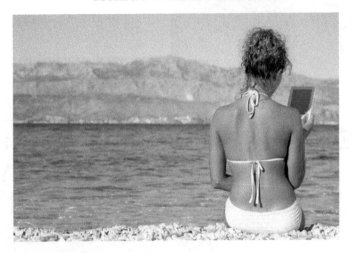

Visit and follow our page and be the first one to find out about new, hot releases as well as free and discounted eBooks dedicated to health, wellness and personal development:

www.YourWellnessBooks.com

Disclaimer

A physician has not written the information in this book. It is advisable that you visit a qualified dietician so that you can obtain a highly personalized treatment for your case, especially if you want to lose weight effectively. This book is for informational and educational purposes only and is not intended for medical purposes. Please consult your physician before making any drastic changes to your diet.

INTRODUCTION

Dear Reader,

Thank you for taking interest in my book. I have written it to show you that eating a healthy Paleo-approved diet is not time-consuming at all. All you need to do is to get committed to it and decide to work on your creativity.

This recipe book is designed to help you become more creative and show you that Paleo salads are not only healthy and delicious but also exciting and fun to prepare.

This book is a great choice for everyone-yes everyone- no matter where you live, how old you are and what you do. Even if you are a vegan, you can benefit from this book, as I have also added a meat-free recipe section. The Paleo Diet is not only about consuming massive amounts of meat. I am not a scientist, but I believe that Paleo cavemen would eat whatever they could find. I am sure they would very often survive long periods of time just munching on fruit, nuts and veggies.

Here's my personal belief that you may agree or disagree with. Even though I am not a vegan or vegetarian, I really do try to eat less and less meat. I think it's healthier and better for the environment. Even if you are a Paleo fan, remember that there is much more to Paleo than just meat.

Of course, you can always change or customize my recipes. I include my e-mail in case you need me to lend you a hand or have problems finding ingredients or are allergic to any of them: elenajamesbooks@gmail.com

This book is especially recommended for:

-Paleo fans

-Alkaline Diet fans (everyone can benefit from adding more fresh fruit and veggies into their diets, right?)

-Health and wellness nuts

-Fitness enthusiasts

-People on weight loss regimes/programs

-Those who wish to detoxify and regain their wellness

-Those who are interested in low-carb diets

WHY I WROTE THIS BOOK

To be honest, I never thought I would write a Paleo recipe book. The reason is simple- I used to be really skeptical about Paleo. I am really passionate about healthy and balanced nutrition though and I love cooking. The diet that I really love (it helped me get healthy and lose weight) is the Alkaline Diet. I still maintain my healthy alkaline balance (70-80% alkaline foods) and I make sure everyone in my family gets used to greens and green smoothies.

However, I like variety as well. My number 1 rule is to go for organic, unprocessed foods and to listen to my body. I would also recommend getting fully committed to healthy cooking, it's not that difficult to learn, especially when it comes to salads.

Ok, so you must be thinking, why is this Alkaline green lady writing a Paleo book?

Well, I want Paleo people to discover more variety- fresh, nutritious, 100% Paleo friendly salad recipes. I also intend to get them hooked on fresh veggies and fruit!

The reason why I was skeptical about Paleo is that I imagined it was only about meat. Then, I began reading and researching and I realized that the true, healthy and balanced Paleo is very similar to the Alkaline Diet (not very strict one though). For example, you can reduce meat to 20% of your diet or even less and make the remaining 80% fresh, alkaline foods. That way you can be both Alkaline and Paleo. My husband and I wrote a bestselling book on how to do it (with practical steps and recipes) and if you are looking for more healthy and balanced nutritional ideas you will love the Alkaline-Paleo mix.

This book could be also approved by most Alkaline (non-vegetarian kind of alkalarians) people: the recipes are abundant in fresh fruit and veggies.

Both Alkaline Diet and Paleo Diet disapprove of bread (gluten products are not on the Alkaline Diet or Paleo Diet) and animal products like milk.

Here are the benefits of eating a Paleo Diet that is also abundant in alkalizing fruits and veggies:

You will detoxify your body and lose weight

You will improve your mental focus and concentrate better

You will restore your energy levels naturally, there will be no need to indulge in caffeine (topic for another book)

By eliminating gluten and processed foods as well as adding more fresh salads you will create a natural anti-inflammatory diet. As a result, your immune system will feel stronger doing a better job for you. Pain, inflammation, even headaches and PMS will be reduced.

Feeling skeptical?

I encourage you to do a little challenge- have at least 1 big bowl of salad a day. Salads are great for a quick-prep lunch. You can also make them to take to work. Fruit salads are a natural source of fiber and vitamins and a great way to reduce sugar cravings. Feeling like sugar? Go for a delicious, fruity, raw Paleo salad. This is going to be a much healthier treat! Plus your energy levels will skyrocket.

Ever since I switched to a natural, Paleo-Alkaline inspired approach and regained balance, I have been able to achieve my perfect weight without thinking too much about it. I don't know about you, but I found calorie counting pretty stressful.

There is also a bonus chapter where I show you how to make amazing, Paleo friendly salsas. Eliminating processed condiments is a must. I know many people who invest time and effort in buying organic greens, but they spoil all their work with artificial condiments.

Mini disclaimer:

Some ingredients suggested (like for example apple cider vinegar and other vinegars) are not Paleo, however many Paleo experts approve them in small amounts. It's up to you if you choose to do strick Paleo-Paleo, or modern Paleo (still healthy and natural).

By switching to natural, home-made salsas and other condiments, you will be able to save up money and make your salads more unique.

Happy salad-ing!

Enjoy!

Before we dive into the recipes, I would like to offer you a free gift...

Alkaline Paleo Newsletter

Join our exclusive Alkaline Paleo newsletter and start receiving the best information on health & wellness from Holistic Wellness Books! You will be the first one to be notified about our new books, eBooks and audiobooks + massive discounts (and even some surprise giveaways). In fact, as soon as you subscribe, you will receive a free copy of our bestselling book: *Alkaline Paleo Superfoods!*

VISIT www.YourWellnessBooks.com/newsletter

to subscribe and get free instant access to this bonus eBook:

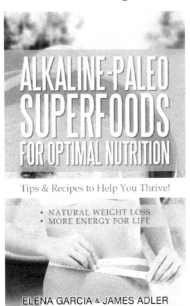

SECTION 1 NO MEAT PALEO SALADS

1. Thai Kale Salad

Servings: 6-7

Preparation time: 15-17 minutes

Cooking time: 2 minutes

Ingredients:

- 1½ lbs. (680 grams) of uncooked kale leaves, stemmed
- 1 large sized red onion, thinly sliced
- Coconut aminos (2 tablespoons)
- Juice of 2 limes
- ½ cup organic coconut milk
- 2 jalapeño peepers, diced
- Zest of 1 lime
- 2 orange sweet peppers, diced
- 3 cloves garlic, peeled, thinly sliced)
- Olive oil (about 2-3 tablespoons)

Method of preparation:

1. Sauté the red onion slices in some olive oil. Add the garlic clove, sweet peppers and jalapeño slices to the onions. Stir-fry until fragrant.
2. Blanch the kale leaves in a pot of boiling water for 2 minutes. Drain and set aside.
3. Mix the coconut aminos, lime zest and lime juice with the coconut milk. Set aside.

4. Toss the kale leaves with the sautéed vegetables and drizzle the coconut milk dressing on top to serve.
5. Enjoy!

2. Apple and Celery Root Salad

Servings: 2-3

Preparation time: 10-15 minutes

Cooking time: 2 hours

Ingredients:

- 1 medium red apple, (skin-on is optional), diced
- 2 tablespoons of Paleo mayonnaise*
- 1 medium sized celery root, peeled and grated
- 4 tablespoons of chopped walnuts
- Paleo Gremolade (2 teaspoons)
- Juice of 1 lemon
- 2 fresh scallions, sliced
- 2 tablespoons of coconut cream
- 1/4th cup of minced fresh parsley leaves

Method of preparation:

1. Toss celery root with diced apples and lemon juice. Then add-in the scallions, walnuts and parsley. Toss again to combine.
2. Mix the gremolade and mayonnaise with coconut yoghurt in another bowl.
3. Add the mayonnaise salad dressing to the apples mixture and then toss to combine.
4. Cover the salad bowl with saran wrap. Store in a fridge for a couple of hours. Serve chilled.

*How to make Paleo Mayo (non-vegan option)

Mix: 1 egg yolk with a pinch of Himalaya salt, half teaspoon of Dijon mustard, 1 tablespoon of lemon juice and a few drops of white vinegar and half cup of avocado oil or coconut oil. Enjoy!

*How to make Paleo Mayo (vegan option)

Mix: half cup almond or coconut milk, 2 tablespoons fresh lemon juice, 1 tablespoon Dijon mustard, half cup of olive oil, pinch of salt and pepper. You can experiment with the consistency by adding some almond powder and coconut oil. Enjoy!

3. Really Simply Kale Caesar Salad with Artichoke Hearts and Pickled Red Onions

Servings: 4-5

Preparation time: 10 minutes

Ingredients:

- 2-3 brine dipped artichoke hearts, halved
- 2 cups of fresh kale leaves, stemmed and coarsely chopped
- Half cup of almond powder mixed with cashew powder (our vegan "parmesan cheese")
- 1 pickled red onion, sliced

Ingredients for the Caesar Dressing:

- 2/3rd cup of homemade mayonnaise (paleo) (check the recipe from the previous recipes)
- 1 garlic clove, peeled and minced
- 6 whole anchovy filets
- Olive oil (3 tablespoons)
- Juice of 1 big lemon

Method of preparation:

1. Mix all the salad ingredients in a big bowl. Set aside.
2. Blend all the ingredients for the salsa.
3. Mix with the salad, stir well and enjoy!

4. Samphire Roast Lemon and Hazelnut Salad

Servings: 2-3

Preparation time: 10-15 minutes

Cooking time: 20 minutes

Ingredients:

- 6.349 oz. (180 grams) of Samphire
- Organic maple syrup, (2 teaspoons)
- 0.881 oz. (25 grams) of hazelnuts
- 1 whole lemon, sliced
- 3 whole radishes
- Olive oil (about 2 tablespoons)

SALAD SALSA

- 1 tablespoon of maple syrup
- 2 tablespoons olive oil,
- Fresh juice of half a lemon
- 2 tablespoons of finely chopped fresh mint leaves

Method of preparation:

1. Preheat an oven to 446 degrees Fahrenheit. Slice lemon into thin slices.

2. Mix the olive oil with the maple syrup (use a bowl). Dip the lemon slices in the maple syrup mixture. Then put on a parchment paper lined baking tray.
3. Insert the tray in the oven and roast for 20 minutes or until the lemon slices start to brown.
4. Mix olive oil, maple syrup and lemon juice. Whisk well to combine and then add-in the mint leaves to prepare the dressing.
5. Lay the hazelnuts in a baking tray and roast for 5 minutes.
6. Steam the samphire for 1 minute over a steamer in the meantime and then rinse the leaves under cold water. Drain properly and set aside.
7. Finally, toss the steamed samphire leaves with the roasted lemon slices and hazelnuts. Drizzle the seasoning on top and to serve. Enjoy!

5. Carpaccio of Summer Veggies

Servings: 4

Preparation time: 20-30 minutes

Ingredients:

- 1 red organic beetroot, peeled and sliced
- 6 whole radishes, sliced
- 1 orange beetroot, peeled and sliced
- 1/2 of a red onion, peeled and sliced
- 2 small courgettes, (zucchini) sliced
- 1 small sized kohlrabi, sliced
- 1 red pepper, deseeded and sliced
- ¼ cup of almonds

Dressing:

- 3 fl. oz. (90 ml) of olive oil (extra virgin)
- 2 teaspoons of fresh oregano, chopped
- 1 clove of garlic, peeled and finely chopped
- 1 teaspoon of organic maple syrup
- 1 tablespoon of fresh parsley leaves, chopped
- 1 tablespoon of water
- Fresh juice of 1 lemon
- Sea salt (a pinch)

Method of preparation:

1. To make the dressing, whisk 3 fl.oz. of olive oil with water, 1 clove of chopped garlic and maple syrup. Then add lemon juice, sea salt, parsley and oregano. Whisk again to combine. Set aside in a fridge while you are preparing the salad.
2. Mix the sliced veggies in a big bowl. Add some almonds and drizzle the salad dressing on top to serve the salad.

6. *Green Papaya Salad*

Servings: 2

Preparation time: 15 minutes

Ingredients:

- 1.763 oz. (50g) of mixed fresh lettuce leaves
- ½ of a green papaya, julienned
- 1 whole radish, sliced
- ½ of a small carrot, julienned
- 2 tablespoons of raw cashew nuts
- A few whole cherry tomatoes, quartered

For the Chilli Spicy Dressing:

- 1 tablespoon of raw coconut vinegar
- 1 tablespoon of raw organic honey
- 2 tablespoons of water
- 1 red long chili, seeded and finely chopped
- Juice of 2 limes
- ½ tablespoon of paleo fish sauce (optional but I suggest you give it a try)
- 1 small clove of garlic, peeled and minced

Method of preparation:

1. Toss the julienned carrots and papaya with radish and lettuce leaves. Transfer the carrots to a salad bowl.

2. Top with the quartered cherry tomatoes and cashews. Set aside.
3. In a separate bowl take the chili slices and other dressing ingredients listed above. Whisk to combine. Set aside in a fridge (optional- depends on your time really)
4. Now mix the salad with the dressing so that all ingredients are equally covered.
5. Serve with some lemon wedges. Enjoy!

7. Grilled Zucchini Salad

Servings: 4

Preparation time: 15-20 minutes

Cooking time: 10-12 minutes

Ingredients:

- 4 whole fresh zucchini, quartered lengthwise
- 1.5 cup of cherry tomatoes, quartered or halved
- 2 tablespoons of sweet onion, minced
- 2 teaspoons of olive oil (extra virgin)
- 8 kalamata olives, pitted and roughly chopped
- A pinch of crashed garlic
- 1 tablespoon of fresh lemon thyme
- 1 tablespoon of fresh dill, chopped
- 1 teaspoon of Dijon mustard (optional)
- Pinch of Himalaya salt
- 1/4th teaspoon black pepper
- Juice from 1/2 a lemon
- 1-2 tablespoons of avocado oil
- Sea salt, according to taste
- Black pepper, to taste

Method of preparation:

1. Toss the zucchini quartered slices in 2 teaspoons of olive oil, salt, garlic, and a bit of black pepper.
2. Set aside and allow the zucchini slices to marinade for 10 minutes.

3. Grill over medium heat once marinating is done until the zucchini slices are charred a bit.
4. Remove from grill once done and let it cool down.
5. Slice the zucchini and set aside.
6. In the meantime, mix some olive oil with mustard and lemon juice. You can mix them directly in a big bowl.
7. Add the cherry tomatoes, olives and sweet onion slices to the zucchini and then toss the vegetables with the olive oil mustard mixture you have just prepared. I sometimes throw in a few raisins, but this is optional.
8. Finally add the chopped herbs and toss again. Serve and enjoy!

8. Summer Slaw with Tahini Coconut Dressing

Servings: 4

Preparation time: 30 minutes

Cooking time: 10-15 minutes

Ingredients for slaw:

- 1 head of fennel, cored and sliced
- 1/4th cup of raisins
- 1/4th of a head of purple cabbage, cored and sliced
- 1/4 cup of Thai basil
- 1 whole bell pepper (yellow colored), seeded and sliced

Ingredients for the dressing:

- 2 tablespoons of fresh coconut milk
- 2 tablespoons of paleo tahini
- 1 inch of fresh ginger, grated (you can also use 1-2 teaspoons of ginger powder)
- 1 teaspoon of paleo raw honey
- Juice of 1 lime
- Pinch of Himalaya Salt
- Pinch of Black pepper

Ingredients for curried cashews:

- 1 cup of raw cashew nuts
- 1/4th teaspoon of paprika
- 1 tablespoon of raw coconut oil
- 1 tablespoon of lime juice
- 1 ½ teaspoons of paleo curry powder
- 1/4th teaspoon of chili powder
- 1/4th teaspoon of turmeric powder

Method of preparation:

1. To prepare the cashews, heat up 1 tablespoon coconut oil in a pan and add the lemon juice and herbs to the oil. Stir fry for a minute and then drop the cashews in the oil.
2. Stir the nuts in the oil for a minute and transfer to a parchment paper lined cookie sheet.
3. Bake the nuts in a 350 degrees preheated oven for 10-15 minutes or unless the nuts turn golden brown in color and crispy. Remove once done and let cool.

4. To prepare the slaw, toss the chopped fennel with cabbage, basil leaves and yellow pepper slices.
5. Whisk all the added ingredients needed to prepare the dressing until a smooth dressing is formed.
6. Drizzle the dressing over the salad and drop the raisins and cashew nuts on top to serve.

9. Beet Salad with Toasted Almonds

Servings: 4

Preparation time: 5-10 minutes

Cooking time: 1 hour

Ingredients:

- 4 whole cooked beets, peeled and sliced
- 1/2 cup of cashew powder
- 2 cups of frisee
- 1 tablespoon of coconut oil
- 1 large apple, cored and sliced thinly
- 1/4th cup olive oil
- 8 tablespoons of almonds
- Sea salt or Himalaya salt to taste

Method of preparation:

1. Boil the beets after trimming their heads. Once boiling, reduce the heat and simmer for about half an hour. Once done, drain and transfer the beets to sink and let sit under cold running water.
2. Once cold, peel off skins of beets and chop into bite sized pieces.
3. Toast the almonds over medium heat for 5 minutes in coconut oil; set aside.
4. Take the beets in a salad bowl and add the frisee, toasted almonds and apple slices. Toss well.
5. Finally toss with sea salt and olive oil. Serve with powdered cashews.

10. Raw Broccoli Slaw

Servings: 4

Preparation time: 10-15 minutes

Cooking time: 10-15 minutes

Ingredients:

- Shredded carrots (1 cup)
- ½ cup of fresh red cherries
- 1½ cups of broccoli florets, shredded
- 3/4th cup of red cabbage, shredded
- ½ cup of thinly sliced red onion
- 1 cup of baby kale leaves

Dressing:

- 3 teaspoons of chia seeds
- 3 teaspoons of Dijon mustard
- 6 tablespoons of coconut vinegar
- 6 tablespoons of extra virgin olive oil
- 1/4th cup of raw honey
- 1/4th teaspoon of freshly crackled black pepper
- ½ teaspoon of koshersalt

Method of preparation:

1. Process the carrots and broccoli florets in a food processor to shred those. Transfer to a large sized salad bowl.

2. Add the onion slices, cherries, kale leaves and shredded red cabbage.
3. Prepare the dressing by mixing everything in a separate bowl.
4. Drizzle the dressing over the slaw and toss before serving.

11. *Rainbow Salad*

Servings: 4-5

Preparation time: 10-15 minutes

Ingredients:

- 1 whole cucumber, diced without peeling
- 1 teaspoon of Dijon mustard (optional)
- 3/4 cup of purple cabbage, chopped
- ½ teaspoon of onion powder
- 1 tablespoon of coconut vinegar
- 2 teaspoons of raw organic honey
- 1 medium sized ripe tomato, diced
- 1 teaspoon of dill
- A pinch of garlic sea salt
- A pinch of ground black pepper

Method of preparation:

1. Chop the vegetables (cabbage, tomato and cucumber) and mix in a bowl.
2. Add the dressing and mix well.
3. Serve the salad right away.

12. Creamy Yummy Broccoli Salad

Servings: 4-6

Preparation time: 20-25 minutes

Ingredients:

- 4 cups of broccoli florets, chopped and steamed
- 1/2 cup of green olives, sliced
- 1/4 cup of pecans, chopped
- 2 mini seedless cucumbers, peeled and diced
- Half cup of raisins
- 4 tablespoons raw coconut vinegar
- 4 cups chopped baby spinach leaves
- 1/2 cup of paleo homemade mayonnaise of your choice (check the previous recipes)
- Juice of 1/2 a lemon
- 1 yellow bell pepper, finely chopped
- 1 orange bell pepper, finely chopped
- 1/2 of a red apple, julienned
- 1 whole red bell pepper, finely chopped
- 1/4 teaspoon of Himalayan salt
- 1/2 teaspoon of black pepper
- 2 slices of lemon or lime to garnish

Method of preparation:

1. Chop the broccoli florets, bell peppers, baby spinach leaves, green olives and cucumbers and set aside in a bowl. Add the rest of the ingredients.
2. Finally sprinkle over the dressing and stir well. Season with salt and pepper to taste.

3. Garnish with a slice of lime or lemon.
4. Enjoy!

13. *Spaghetti Squash Yoga Bowl*

Servings: 4

Preparation time: 20 minutes

Cooking time: 10 minutes

Ingredients:

- 2 bunches of small broccoli
- 2 lbs. (907 grams) of spaghetti squash
- 1 tablespoon of coconut oil
- 4 kale stalks
- Cashew nuts
- Sesame seeds
- Red pepper flakes

Sauce:

- Coconut aminos (2 tablespoons)
- 2-3 medium garlic cloves
- 1 tablespoon of coconut sugar
- 1 tablespoon of coconut vinegar
- 2 tablespoons raw cashew butter
- 1 1-inch piece of fresh ginger, peeled and grated
- 1/3 cup coconut oil
- 1 whole lime
- 1/2 tablespoon of Himalaya salt
- 1 tablespoon of sesame oil

Method of preparation:

1. Cook the spaghetti squash until thoroughly cooked. Remove the spaghetti squash from the heat and let it cool down.
2. Scrape and extract the flesh of the squash.
3. To prepare the sauce for the salad, process all the sauce ingredients in a food processor.
4. Process to get a smooth salad sauce. Set the sauce aside in a bowl once done.
5. Toss the spaghetti squash with the salad sauce and set aside.
6. Chop the broccoli florets and set those aside in a bowl.
7. Heat up 1 tablespoon of coconut oil in a skillet and stir-fry the broccoli florets. Keep stir-frying until slightly brownish.
8. Then add the kale leaves and cook those for a few more minutes. Make sure the kale leaves start to wilt. Finally add-in the spaghetti squash and cook for a few more seconds until cooked through.
9. Serve the salad with cashew nuts, red pepper flakes or sesame seeds. Enjoy!

14. Spinach Almonds and Tomatoes Salad

Servings: 4

Preparation time: 10-15 minutes

Cooking time: 15-20 minutes

Ingredients:

- 1/2 cup of almonds
- 2 cups of baby spinach
- 2 big carrots, peeled and sliced
- 15 cherry tomatoes
- 1 teaspoon of red chili flakes
- 2 teaspoons of sumac
- 2 medium garlic cloves (peeled and chopped)
- 1 tablespoon of olive oil
- A pinch of Himalaya sea salt

Method of preparation:

1. Toast the almonds in some olive oil. Stir to mix and set aside to allow it to cool down the almonds.
2. Then, stir-fry the garlic and red pepper. Add the tomatoes once the garlic is slightly browned. Cook until the tomatoes start releasing their juices.
3. Finally add the sumac and the toasted almonds to the tomato mixture. Stir the mixture to combine well. Cool it down and mix with spinach and carrots. Store in a fridge for about 15 minutes. Add a bit of Himalaya salt and olive oil to taste. Serve and enjoy!

15. Salad Savoy

Servings: 4-5

Preparation time: 15-20 minutes

Cooking time: 15-17 minutes

Ingredients:

- ½ cup of shiitake mushrooms
- 1 bunch of salad savoy cabbage
- 2 tablespoons of vegan cheese (powdered almonds and cashews)
- 1 medium sized red onion, peeled and sliced
- 1 medium sized clementine, peeled and segmented
- 2 cloves garlic (peeled, minced)
- 4 stalks of asparagus, cut into ribbons
- 1 tablespoon of coconut butter

Ingredients for dressing:

- 1 lemon, juiced
- Sea salt, to taste
- 2 tablespoons of olive oil
- A dash of grated ginger

Method of preparation:

1. Melt the coconut butter in a skillet and dump the onion and garlic slices to the oil.

2. Sauté the onions and garlic until softened and translucent in color. Once that happens, add the asparagus ribbons and shiitake mushrooms to the onion mixture in the skillet.
3. Then add the salad savoy to the mixture and cook the mushrooms mixture lid-on on low heat for 5 minutes.
4. Remove the lid from the skillet, give stir the mixture lightly and cook the mixture again without lid for 10 minutes on low heat.
5. Finally add the vegan Paleo cheese and the clementine segments to the salad. Give a nice stir to combine, turn down the heat and let it cool down a bit.
6. In the meantime, blend all the salad ingredients.
7. Toss the salad with the dressing and serve right away. Enjoy!

16. Simple Celery Salad

Servings: 2-3

Preparation time: 10 minutes

Ingredients:

- 1 ½ cups of celery, sliced
- 1 ½ tablespoons of Paleo mayonnaise
- 1 tablespoon of chives (minced)
- 1/2 teaspoon of fresh, organic lemon juice
- Sea salt, to taste
- 3 tablespoons raw raisins
- A pinch of black pepper

Method of preparation:

1. Stir and mix the paleo mayonnaise with lemon juice, sea salt and black pepper using in a salad bowl.
2. Slice the celery and chives. Dump the sliced vegetables and the raisins in the mayonnaise mixture.
3. Stir and toss the salad to coat the vegetables with the mayonnaise dressing and then serve to enjoy.

17. Pistachio Kale Salad

Servings: 4

Preparation time: 20-30 minutes

Ingredients:

- ½ cup of shelled pistachios, roughly chopped
- 2 bunches of dinosaur kale, very thinly sliced
- 4 scallions, very thinly sliced
- ¼ cup of raw sesame seeds

For the salad:

- 1/3 cup of paleo tahini paste
- 1/3 cup of plain water
- 1 garlic clove, peeled
- Sea salt, to taste
- 2 tablespoons of juice of lemon
- 1 tablespoon miso paste

Method of preparation:

1. To prepare the salad dressing, blend all the ingredients until smooth and lightly thick. Add more water or coconut milk to the salad dressing to achieve the right consistency.
2. Cut and chop the vegetables and combine the kale with scallions in a bowl. Pour the salad dressing over the scallion mixture and toss to combine.

3. Finally, sprinkle the sesame seeds and the chopped pistachios on top of the salad to garnish and serve the salad

18. Greek Style Bell Pepper Salad

Servings: 4

Preparation time: 20-25 minutes

Ingredients:

- 1 large orange bell pepper (cut into chunks)
- 1 cup of jumbo Kalamata olives, pitted
- 1 large yellow bell pepper (cut into chunks)
- 2 green onions, chopped
- 1 green bell pepper, cubed
- 1/2 cup of organic walnuts, chopped
- 1 red bell pepper, cut into chunks
- 4 medium Lebanese cucumbers, halved lengthwise, seeded and sliced
- 1/4 cup parsley
- 1/2 lb. (225 grams) of paleo cashew feta cheese, diced

***To make Paleo Cashew Feta Style Cheese, simply blend the following ingredients: 1 cup of raw cashews previously soaked in water for at least a few hours (I leave it to soak overnight and I use alkaline water), about ¼ cup of almond milk or coconut milk, 1 tablespoon of lime juice, ¼ cup of nutritional yeast, 1 clove of garlic and a bit of Himalaya salt to taste. Transfer into little cubes (like for ice making) and store in a fridge for a few hours.

Ingredients for the vinaigrette:

- 1 tablespoon of za'atar
- 1/4th cup of olive oil (extra-virgin)
- 1 tablespoon of dried oregano, organic
- 2 tablespoons of paleo vinegar (white wine)
- 2 large garlic cloves, peeled and minced
- 1/2 teaspoon of Himalayan salt
- 1 tablespoon of sumac
- 1/2 teaspoon fresh black pepper

Method of preparation:

1. Prepare the salad dressing by taking all the ingredients required for the vinaigrette in medium sized bowl. Whisk with a fork or a blender to prepare the dressing.
2. Now peel and chop all the vegetables and transfer to a salad bowl. Drizzle the homemade vinaigrette over the salad. Toss lightly to coat the vegetables with the vinaigrette.
3. Serve the salad as it is or chill for a few hours before serving.

19. Gingered Peas and Cucumber Salad

Servings: 5

Preparation time: 10 minutes

Ingredients:

- 3 Persian cucumbers, peeled and thinly sliced
- 1 tablespoons of grated ginger
- 2 tablespoons of olive oil
- 1 teaspoon of raw honey
- 2 tablespoons of pure organic lemon juice
- 1 shallot, thinly sliced
- Zest of 1 lemon
- Black pepper, to taste
- Sea salt, to taste

Method of preparation:

1. Slice the shallots and cucumbers. Set aside the chopped vegetables in a salad bowl.
2. Now combine the lemon zest, grated ginger, lemon juice, black pepper, olive oil and sea salt. Mix well and add to the salad. Serve right away. Enjoy!

20. Cucumber and Radish Salad

Servings: 5-6

Preparation time: 20-25 minutes

Ingredients:

- 1 whole cucumber, thinly sliced
- 3 stems of parsley leaves, stemmed and chopped
- 7 whole radishes, sliced thinly
- Sea salt, to taste
- 2 tablespoons raw coconut vinegar
- ½ of a red onion, peeled and sliced thinly
- 2 tablespoons of olive oil
- Black pepper, to taste

Method of preparation:

1. Slice the radishes, cucumber and onion. Set aside the sliced vegetables in a bowl.
2. Remove the leaves from the parsley stems and add those to the sliced vegetables in the bowl.
3. Now add the coconut vinegar, sea salt, olive oil and ground black pepper to salad. Mix well. Enjoy!

SECTION 2 FISH-Y PALEO SALADS

21. *Two Minutes Tuna Salad*

It takes only a couple of minutes to prepare, but you need much more time to drool over it!

Servings: 2-3

Preparation time: 2-3 minutes

Ingredients:

- 1 can of paleo albacore tuna, drained
- 2 tablespoons of cashew nuts
- 1/4 cup of chopped tomatoes
- 2 cups of baby spinach
- 2-3 tablespoons of homemade paleo pesto (simply blend some olive oil with Himalaya salt and fresh basil leaves and tomato juice)
- 1/4 cup of chopped bell peppers

Method of preparation:

1. Take drained tuna in a bowl. Add the bell peppers, spinach, cashew nuts and tomatoes to the tuna.
2. Toss the drained tuna mixture with pesto. Serve.
3. Enjoy!

22. *Confetti Rice Salad with Salmon*

Servings: 2

Preparation time: 5-10 minutes

Ingredients:

- 1 cup of steamed cauliflower rice
- 3-4 oz. (113.4 grams) of cooked salmon
- 1/3rd cup of artichoke hearts
- 4 teaspoons of paleo mayonnaise
- 2 teaspoons of toasted cashew nuts
- 4 teaspoons of paleo white balsamic vinegar
- 1 cup celery, finely sliced
- 1 teaspoon of extra virgin olive oil
- 1/3rd cup of thinly sliced red or orange bell peppers
- 1/4th teaspoon of dry thyme
- 1.5 teaspoons of curry powder
- 11 whole scallion, sliced
- A pinch of Himalaya salt
- Fresh ground black pepper, according to taste

Method of preparation:

1. Whisk together thyme, paleo mayonnaise, balsamic vinegar, curry powder, olive oil and a pinch of salt. Set aside.
2. Add the scallions, artichoke hearts, bell pepper slices, celery slices, salmon and cashews with the cauliflower rice.
3. Add the mayonnaise dressing and toss again before serving to make sure it's equally spread on all the ingredients. Enjoy!

23. *Apple Pecan Tuna Salad*

Servings: 2-3

Preparation time: 10 minutes

Ingredients:

- 1 can of drained tuna
- 3 tablespoons of pecans
- 1/2 an apple, diced
- 1-2 tablespoons coconut yogurt
- 1/2 a stalk of celery, diced
- Ground black pepper, as required
- 1/2 lemon, juiced
- Sea salt, to taste

Method of preparation:

1. Chop the fruits and vegetables as is instructed and put in a bowl.
2. Add the remaining ingredients and stir well to combine. Serve and enjoy! I love coconut yoghurt or coconut milk (a nice alternative if you can't find coconut yoghurt) in my salads!

24. *Quick Salmon Salad*

Servings: 2-3

Preparation time: 10-15 minutes

Ingredients:

- 1 can of wild caught salmon, drained
- 1/4 cup of radicchio, shredded
- 1/4 cup of raw walnuts, chopped
- 1/2 ripe avocado (peeled and diced)
      3.5oz. (100g) mixed leafy greens
- 4 tablespoons of paleo mayo
- 1 medium sized endive, sliced
- 3 oz. (85g) of baby spinach leaves, roughly chopped
- 2 tablespoons of lemon juice
- 3 large sized mushrooms, stemmed and sliced
- 1 small seedless cucumber, diced
- 1/2 teaspoon of freshly cracked black pepper
- 1 teaspoon of herbes de Provence
- 1/4 teaspoon of Himalayan or sea salt
- 2 tablespoons of olive oil

Method of preparation:

1. Dump everything into a salad bowl after chopping and slicing as necessary. Mix well.
2. Season the salad with Himalayan salt, pepper, olive oil, lemon juice and toss well to combine.
3. Sprinkle the remaining salmon on top to serve.

25. *Creamy Tarragon Tuna Apple Salad*

Servings: 2

Preparation time: 10 minutes

Ingredients:

- 2 small sized cans of wild tuna
- 1/2 of an English cucumber, peeled and finely chopped
- 1 whole apple, cored and chopped
- Honeyed Walnuts (optional)
- 2 whole scallions, minced

Ingredients for dressing:

- 4 tablespoons of paleo mayo
- 3 tablespoons of tarragon, minced
- 1 small clove of garlic
- Sea salt, to taste
- 1 tablespoons of fresh lemon juice
- Pinch of black pepper

Method of preparation:

1. To prepare the salad, empty the tuna can into a large salad bowl. Add the remaining ingredients and stir well to combine.
2. Prepare the dressing by mixing the ingredients for the dressing in a separate bowl.

3. Pour the salad dressing over the salad, toss lightly and serve. Enjoy!

26. Salmon Arugula Salad with Lemon Parsley Dressing

Servings: 4

Preparation time: 40 minutes

Ingredients:

- 1 lb. (453 g) of grilled salmon fillets
- 1 whole scallion, finely chopped
- 4 cups of fresh arugula, chopped
- Fresh chopped parsley for topping
- 1 whole ripe avocado, peeled, pitted and cubed
- 2 tablespoons of capers (optional)

For the dressing:

- 2 tablespoons of extra virgin olive oil
- 4 tablespoons of parsley, chopped
- 2 tablespoons organic lemon juice
- Sea salt
- A pinch of pepper
- Lemon wedges, for garnishing

Method of preparation:

1. Cut the cooked or grilled salmon filets into bite sized pieces and place in a bowl.
2. Chop the vegetables as mentioned.

3. Combine everything with the salmon pieces except for the fresh parsley. Toss to mix and transfer the bowl to a refrigerator to let the salad sit there for 30 minutes.
4. In the meantime, prepare the salad dressing by mixing all the salad dressing ingredients (use a small bowl). Set aside.
5. Once the salad is cooled down, drizzle the dressing on top.
6. Toss the salad to mix the dressing and then finally sprinkle fresh parsley on top to serve. Enjoy!

27. Poached Cod and Citrus Salad

Servings: 2

Preparation time: 8-10 minutes

Cooking time: 4-5 minutes

Ingredients:

- 2 fresh filets of cod
- Juice of 1 lemon
- 1 whole fennel bulb with the stalks
- 1/2 tablespoons of olive oil
- 1/2 teaspoon of fennel leaves
- 1 medium-sized sweet tangelo or orange or blood orange, peeled and sliced
- A pinch of sea salt

Method of preparation:

1. Bring a pot of water to boil. In the meantime, cut the fennel bulb into thin slices. Set aside.
2. Mix the olive oil with fennel leaves, sea salt and lemon juice. Set aside.
3. Once water starts boiling, drop the cod filets in the water and poach for 4-5 minutes until the filets turn opaque and flaky in nature. Cool to cut into bite sized pieces.
4. Slice the citrus fruit after peeling it. Slice the fruit horizontally to get wheel-like slices.
5. Toss the fennel bulb slices with citrus slices and cod pieces. Drizzle lemon juice dressing on top and toss again to serve. Enjoy!

28.Keto Tuna Salad

Servings: 2-3

Preparation time: 5 times

Cooking time: 8-10 minutes

Ingredients:

- 1 3.5-oz. (100g) head of lettuce, (Little Gem or Romaine)
- 2 tablespoons of paleo mayonnaise (preferably homemade) 6oz. (180g) of organic tuna, drained
- Juice from 1/4th of a lemon
- 2 hard-boiled eggs, free-range
- A bit of olive oil
- 1 0.5-oz. (15g) medium sized spring onion
- Himalayan salt, to taste

Method of preparation:

1. Hard boil the eggs and then cut those in halves. Line salad bowl with the lettuce leaves.
2. Place the egg halves all over the lettuce leaves, so as to place an egg half over one lettuce leaf. Toss the tuna pieces in the lemon juice before placing over the lettuce leaves.
3. Drizzle the mayonnaise and extra virgin olive oil over the salad and serve.

29 Nicoise Salad

Servings: 2-3

Preparation time: 20 minutes

Cooking time: 15-20 minutes

Ingredients:

- 8 oz. (226.79 grams) of organic tuna steak, seared
- 1 pint of fresh cherry tomatoes
- 2-3 tablespoons of whole Niçoise olives, pitted
- 1 whole medium potato (boiled and pan sautéed in coconut oil)
- 1-2 eggs, poached
- 2 cups of spinach
- 4-6 filets of anchovies
- 8-10 leaves of butter lettuce
- 2-3 teaspoons of caper berries
- A pinch (or 2) of garlic powder
- Coconut oil, for cooking

For dressing:

- 3 tablespoons of Dijon mustard
- 1/2 tablespoon of organic olive oil
- Sea salt, to taste
- 1 tablespoon of coconut vinegar
- Black pepper, to taste

Method of preparation:

1. Boil the whole potatoes until slightly soft. Cut the boiled potatoes into slices and then sauté those in the coconut oil until crisp and set aside.
2. Add the spinach and stir-fry in using the same coconut oil mixed with garlic powder, add more oil if needed.
3. Add the tuna steaks and stir-fry so that they absorb coconut oil taste. Turn off the heat and set aside and let it cool down. The spinach will have an incredible taste!
4. To arrange the salad, lay the lettuce leaves flat on a salad platter and then arrange the eggs sunny side up. Arrange the rest of the salad as desired.
5. Finally, whisk all the ingredients of the dressing and drizzle over salad before serving. Enjoy!

30.Tuna with Roasted Broccoli Salad

Servings: 1-2

Preparation time: 20 minutes

Cooking time: 30-35 minutes

Ingredients:

- 2-3 cups of roasted broccoli, chopped into florets
- 6-8 pieces of whole green olives
- 5 oz. (141.7 grams) of wild caught tuna, drained
- 1/2 of a whole avocado, peeled and mashed
- 5 fresh cherry tomatoes, quartered
- 1/3 cup of almonds
- A pinch of sea salt
- 1 tablespoon of paleo Dijon mustard
- 1 tablespoon of olive oil
- 1-2 oz. of paleo feta cheese, diced (Optional)
- Black pepper, to taste

Method of preparation:

1. Chop the broccoli into florets and transfer to a baking dish. Drizzle over some olive oil.
2. Add the dried garlic, salt and black pepper to the broccoli florets.
3. Toss the broccoli florets with the added ingredients and transfer to a 400 degrees Fahrenheit preheated oven. Roast for 30-35 minutes.
4. Mix the tuna with the Dijon mustard, a pinch of sea salt and mashed avocado. Set aside.

5. Sauté the broccoli florets in some oil until crisp. Add the paleo vegan cheese to the pan and allow it to melt in the pan over the broccoli florets.
6. Set aside to cool down.
7. Toss the tuna with the broccoli florets and then add a little bit of olive oil, the almonds and the quartered cherry tomatoes to the mixture.
8. Toss the mixture to prepare the salad. Serve chilled. Enjoy!

31. *Lemon Salmon Salad*

Servings: 1-2

Preparation time: 5-8 minutes

Ingredients:

- 1 piece of cooked salmon darne, roughly chopped
- Flaked almonds
        3.5oz. (100g) of spinach
- 6 pieces of sun-dried tomatoes, finely diced
- Juice from 1/4th lemon
- 2 tablespoons of powdered nuts
- 2 tablespoons of sliced scallions

Method of preparation:

1. Cut salmon darne pieces into bite sized pieces.
2. Toss all the other ingredients with the salmon and serve.
3. You can use your dinner leftovers and conjure up and incredibly healthy and energizing Paleo friendly salad for lunch or even for breakfast! Full-on energy!

32. Chopped Salad with Tuna

Servings: 2-3

Preparation time: 15 minutes

Cooking time: 5 minutes

Ingredients:

- 6-oz. (170 grams) of fresh water-packed tuna, wild caught and drained
- 1 celery stalk, chopped
- ½ cup of chopped radishes
- 1 whole cucumber,chopped
- 1 cup of chopped romaine lettuce
- 1 medium sized tomato, chopped
- 1 whole avocado, peeled, pitted and diced
- 1 carrot, chopped
- For the Dressing:
- 2 garlic cloves, minced
- 3 teaspoons of olive oil
- A pinch of Himalaya salt
- 2 tablespoons of fresh lime juice
- ½ teaspoon of ground black pepper

Method of preparation:

1. Place all the veggies in a salad bowl, cover and set aside.
2. Combine the dressing ingredients in another bowl. Finally, combine tuna with the salad in the bowl and toss lightly to mix.

3. Then drizzle the salad dressing over the vegetables and tuna salad and serve right away. Enjoy!

33.Avocado Codfish Salad

Servings: 5-6

Preparation time: 15-20 minutes

Cooking time: 1 hour

Ingredients:

- 1 Packet of organic salted codfish, boneless
- 1 whole avocado, pitted and diced
- 1 tomato, peeled, halved and sliced
- 1/2 teaspoon of adobo sauce (some experts say it's not really Paleo, so let's make it optional, unless you don't mind minor cheatings here and there)
- 1 red onion, peeled and chopped
- 2 fresh limes, juiced
- 2 teaspoons of olive oil
- Jalapeno
- 1 teaspoon of black pepper
- 1 teaspoon kosher salt
- A handful of chopped cilantro

Method of preparation:

1. Bring a pot of fresh water to boil and drop the cod fish in it.
2. Boil the fish for half an hour until soft. Once done, drain the water, remove the fish from heat and allow it to cool down. Once the fish cools down, cut it into bite sized squares.
3. Next chop the avocado, cilantro, onion and tomato to get medium sized pieces of vegetables.
4. Place the vegetables in a salad bowl. Add the cod fish pieces to the mixture.

5. Drizzle fresh juice of 2 limes, olive oil and adobo sauce over the salad. Season with kosher salt and black pepper as required and toss the salad to blend the flavors. Serve immediately.

34.Escondido Codfish Salad

Servings: 4

Preparation time: 1 hour 15 minutes

Cooking time: 5-7 minutes

Ingredients:

- 1 lb. (453.6 grams) fillet of fresh codfish
- 1 large green bell pepper (seeded and diced
- ½ lb. (226.8 grams) of jicama (peeled and grated)
- ½ cup of fresh lime juice
- 1 small sized jalapeno chili (seeded and minced)
- ½ cup of fresh lemon juice
- 2 scallions, minced
- 2 tablespoons of paleo coconut vinegar
- 1 tablespoon of lime rind (grated)
- ½ cup of mint leaves
- ½ cup of basil leaves
- 4 tablespoons of olive oil
- 2 whole carrots, peeled, grated
- ½ teaspoon of salt, plus more to taste
- 1 cup of coriander leaves
- 1 teaspoon ground pepper

Method of preparation:

1. Bring a pot full of 1 inch up water to boil.
2. Place a slotted tray over the pot and put the cod fish fillet over the plate.
3. Steam the fish for 5-7 minutes.
4. Once done, cool down the fish in the refrigerator. Once chilled, remove from the refrigerator and shred the fish. Set aside.

5. In a bowl, whisk the lemon juice, sugar, lime rind, jalapeno, salt and lime juice. Add in the olive oil after whisking the lemon juice mixture for a few seconds.
6. Dip the shredded cod fish in the lemon juice mixture and toss. Place back in refrigerator and let refrigerate for 1 hour.
7. Remove from fridge after 1 hour and add all the other remaining ingredients.
8. Toss well and serve the salad.

35. Smoked Mackerel and New Potato Salad

Servings: 2

Preparation time: 15 minutes

Cooking time: 15- 20 minutes

Ingredients:

- 8 oz. (200 grams) of smoked mackerel fillets, skinned and flaked
- 12.34 oz. (350 grams) of new potatoes
- 1 teaspoon of horseradish cream
- 3.5 oz. (100 grams) of coconut yoghurt
- 3 oz. (85 grams) of fresh watercress
- Juice of 1 lemon
- A dash of ground black pepper

Method of preparation:

1. Rinse the potatoes very nicely under running water, as new potatoes tend to have a lot of dirt on them. Rinse the potatoes until the water turns clear and no longer retains the murkiness. Bring a pot of salted water to boil and once the water starts boiling, drop the rinsed new potatoes in the pot. Let the potatoes boil in the water until tender, which will take approximately 15-20 minutes.
2. While the potatoes are boiling, mix up the coconut yoghurt, horseradish cream and fresh lemon juice in a big bowl.
3. Season with some black pepper and stir slightly to combine well and to get a lump free smooth dressing.

70

4. Once the potatoes are cooked, drain them off and cool them down. Then cut them in halves. Leave aside.
5. Add the smoked mackerel and the watercress to the yoghurt dressing and toss. Finally add the halved potatoes and toss again to coat. Serve the warm salad right away.

36. Khmer Fish Salad

Servings: 2

Preparation time: 10 minutes

Ingredients:

- 3oz. (80 grams) of snapper fillet, finely sliced
- A bunch of asparagus, chopped and previously boiled
- 0.881 oz. (25 grams) of white cabbage, thinly sliced
- A handful of fresh mint leaves
- 0.881 oz. (25 grams) of purple cabbage, thinly sliced
- 2 fresh red Asian shallots, thinly sliced
- 0.881 oz. (25 grams) of iceberg lettuce, thinly sliced
- A handful of fresh spinach
- 2 teaspoon of organic raw honey
- 1 Lebanese cucumber, julienned
- 3oz. (80 grams) of green capsicum, thinly sliced
- 1 teaspoon of paleo fish sauce
- A handful of fresh Vietnamese mint leaves
- 1 whole carrot, julienned
- A handful of fresh Thai basil leaves

For the lime marinade:

- 0.405 fl. oz. (12 ml) of fresh lime juice
- A pinch of thinly sliced lemongrass, white part only
- 1 teaspoon of coriander paste
- A pinch of sea salt
- Garnish:
- Sliced red chilies

- Roasted unsalted crushed peanuts

Method of preparation:

1. Slice up all the vegetables (carrot, iceberg lettuce, asparagus, cucumber, purple cabbage, green capsicum, white cabbage and Asian shallots) and dump in a large salad bowl.
2. Now slice the snapper fillet in diagonal sections across the bone and place in a bowl. Add 12 ml of fresh lime juice, coriander paste and thinly sliced lemongrass to the fish slices and give a gentle toss to the mixture. Let the fish marinate in the marinade for 10-12 minutes or until the fish turns its color into opaque white. Once done, strain the fish slices from the marinade and squeeze out all of the marinade from the fish slices. Set the fish slices aside to be used later.
3. Add the spinach and fresh herbs and mix well with the veggies.
4. Now combine the fish slices to the salad and add the fish sauce, honey and the reserved lime marinade to the salad. Toss the entire salad gently a few times and serve straight away.

37. Warm Fish Salad

Servings: 4

Preparation time: 20 minutes

Cooking time: 6-8 minutes

Ingredients:

- 24.69 oz. (700 grams) of white fish fillets, skinless
- 1 medium sized Lebanese cucumber, thinly sliced
- oz. (120 grams) of Asian salad mix
- 1 small sized red capsicum, (remove the seeds and slice)
- 1-2 tablespoons of olive oil, to coat
- 1½ cups of fresh spinach
- 1 small sized carrot, julienned
- For the dressing:
- 2 tablespoons of raw organic honey
- Fresh juice of 1 lemon
- 2 cloves of garlic, thinly chopped
- 1½ tablespoons of paleo fish sauce
- 1 teaspoon of fresh grated ginger
- 1 teaspoon of sesame oil
- 1 small sized red chili, chopped

Method of preparation:

1. Heat up a charcoal grill to moderate heat.
2. Then, slice the fish filets into bite sized (3-4 cm) pieces and dump in a bowl. Drizzle vegetable oil over the fish pieces and toss the pieces to coat those nicely on all sides with the oil.

3. Take a saucepan of hot water and drop the spinach leaves. Blanch for a few minutes and then strain immediately to avoid overcooking.
4. Combine in a bowl all of the dressing ingredients and set aside.
5. Now place the fish slices on the hot prepared grill and grill for approximately 2-3 minutes on each side of the fish or until the fish slices turn tender and develop light grill marks on them.
6. Once done, let the grilled fish cool down a bit and then mix it with the veggies and the dressing. Enjoy!

38.Grilled Fish and Zucchini Salad

Servings: 2

Preparation time: 10 minutes

Cooking time: 30 minutes

Ingredients:

- 2 big zucchini, cut into chunks
- 2 white fish filets
- Olive oil, (1 teaspoon)
- 3 oz. (85 grams) of roasted red peppers, chopped
- 6 pitted black olives
- A bunch of fresh rocket leaves
- 1 large clove of garlic, crushed
- 1 tablespoon of paleo mayonnaise
- A pinch of sea salt
- Ground black, freshly crushed

Method of preparation:

1. Heat up a grill and place a heavy duty foil over the grill. Grease it with some oil.
2. Now take the fish filets and grease those with oil as well. Season the fish filets with salt and pepper and let then place the filets over the hot grill.
3. Let the fish filets sit on the grill for 6-8 minutes or until the fish is cooked all the way through and starts to flake pretty easily.
4. Boil the zucchini (low heat) for 15 minutes until soft. Avoid overcooking. Once done, drain the water from the pot and dump the potatoes in a pan.

5. Stir the olives, crushed garlic and roasted red peppers with the boiled potatoes in the pan. Finally, add-in the paleo mayonnaise and stir lightly to combine.
6. Serve the grilled fish pieces salad over the rocket leaves and the zucchini mixture.

39. Easy Tuna and Spinach Salad

Servings: 4-6

Preparation time: 15 minutes

Ingredients:

- 14 oz. (400 grams) of wild caught fresh tuna fish in oil
- 2 oz. (56.7 grams) red onion, sliced
- 9 oz. (250 g) of radish
- 1 oz. (25 grams) of fresh rocket leaves

For the dressing:

- 2 cloves of garlic, peeled
- 3 tablespoons of fresh lemon juice
- 1 teaspoon mustard powder
- 2 tablespoons of olive oil
- A pinch of salt
- Zest of 1 big lemon
- 1 teaspoon of black peppercorns

Method of preparation:

1. Drain the tuna fish from the oil and reserve the oil. Set aside both the fish pieces and the oil for later use.
2. Press the garlic cloves with sea salt in a mortar and pestle and then add the mustard powder to the mixture. Process again to combine. Grind the peppercorns in as well and then add the lemon juice, 3 tablespoons of reserved tuna oil,

zest of lemon and extra virgin olive oil to the garlic mixture in the mortar. Mix everything up nicely with a spoon to prepare the salad dressing and then keep aside.

3. Coat the rocket leaves with the dressing, make sure all the leaves are nicely covered for optimal taste. Add the rest of the ingredients and top with tuna chunks. Serve immediately, enjoy!

40.Fish Fillets with Cress and Avocado Salad

Servings: 1

Preparation time: 10-15 minutes

Cooking time: 7-8 minutes

Ingredients:

- 6 oz. (170 grams) of white fish fillets, skin removed
- A bunch of watercress
- 1 egg, nicely beaten
- 2 tablespoons of almond flour
- Juice of 1/2 a lemon
- 1/2 of a red chili, deseeded and chopped finely
- 2 oz. (56.7 grams) of almond powder
- 1 whole ripe avocado (peeled, pitted and sliced)
- 1 tablespoon olive oil
- Sea salt
- A pinch of black pepper

Method of preparation:

1. Prepare a frying pan by putting some oil in it. Place the pan on medium high heat.
2. While the pan is getting ready, mix up the almond flour with ground black pepper and sea salt.
3. Beat the egg in another bowl and keep the bowl aside.
4. Take the fish filets and dump those one by one in the almond flour mixture. Coat with the mixture of flour nicely

on all sides and thereafter, transfer the filets immediately to the bowl of the beaten eggs.

5. Dip the fish filets in the egg and then coat with some almond powder. Once done, fry the "paleo cheese"coated fish filets in the heated pan after greasing that with a little bit of oil. Let the filets brown a bit while frying. Add the red chili after a few minutes and stir fry for a few seconds.

6. Toss the watercress and avocado with lemon juice and some olive oil.

7. Put all of these ingredients in a plate and top with the fish filets to serve.

SECTION 3 PALEO CHICKEN SALADS

41. Pink Chicken Salad

Servings: 4

Preparation time: 1 hour

Ingredients:

- 1½ lbs. (680.3 grams) of cooked chicken, shredded
- 3/4 cup of dried cranberries
- 3/4 cup of diced celery
- 2 teaspoons of sea salt
- 2 fresh green onions, diced
- ½ cup of fresh grapes, sliced in half
- 1½ teaspoons of black pepper
- ¾ cup of strained coconut yogurt
- 1 teaspoon of smoked paprika

Method of preparation:

1. Dice and chop the vegetables as required. Transfer all of those to a salad bowl.
2. Mix all the other ingredients and then toss all to combine.
3. Transfer to refrigerator and let chill for 1 hour or more before serving.
4. Serve over home-made paleo gluten free bread or lettuce leaves.

42. Avocado Chicken Salad

Servings: 2-3

Preparation time: 5 minutes

Ingredients:

- 1 lb. (453.592 grams) chicken, cooked and shredded
- 4 tablespoons of onions, finely diced
- 3 whole avocados
- Black pepper
- 1 medium sized fresh tomato, diced
- A pinch of sea salt
- 4 whole limes, juiced

Method of preparation:

1. Peel and pit the avocados and mash those. Add all the other ingredients.
2. Combine the added ingredients with the avocado and serve. Enjoy!

43. Curry Love Chicken Salad

Servings: 6

Preparation time: 10 minutes

Cooking time: 10 minutes

Ingredients:

- 12 oz. (340 grams) of chicken (cooked and diced)
- 6 radicchio cups
- 1 cup of walnut halves
- 1/2 cup of mayonnaise
- 1 cup of red grapes
- 2 tablespoons of coconut vinegar
- 1 large celery rib, halved lengthwise and thinly sliced crosswise
- 2 scallions, trimmed and thinly sliced
- 1/3 cup of coconut vinegar
- 3 oz. (85 grams) of mixed baby greens
- ¼ teaspoon of curry powder
- ¼ teaspoon of black pepper

Method of preparation:

1. Toast the walnuts in a 375 degrees Fahrenheit oven for 10 minutes. Chop coarsely after done.
2. Toss 3/4th of the walnuts with chicken, celery and grapes in a salad bowl.
3. In another bowl, mix the paleo mayonnaise, scallions, curry powder, coconut vinegar and black pepper.
4. Cover the chicken and walnuts with the dressing and toss well.
5. Serve in radicchio cups and sprinkle the greens around it.

44. *Grilled Chicken Salad with Mango and Avocado*

Servings: 4

Preparation time: 15 minutes

Cooking time: 8 minutes

Ingredients:

- 4 skinless chicken breast halves (remove the bones)
- 2 tablespoons of mango chutney
- 8 cups of mixed salad greens
- 2 tablespoons of olive oil
- 1 cup of peeled and diced mango
- 2 tablespoons of fresh lime juice
- 3/4th cup of avocado, peeled and diced
- 1 tablespoon of coconut aminos
- Cooking spray
- 3/4th teaspoon of grated fresh ginger

Method of preparation:

1. Preheat a grill and grease it with some cooking spray.
2. Take a bowl and combine the coconut aminos, chutney, lime juice, olive oil and ginger in it. Keep aside.
3. Lay the chicken breast halves on a flat surface and brush those with 2 tablespoons of the chutney mixture.
4. Grill the chicken for 4 minutes on each side while coating lightly with the chutney mixture again on flipping. Remove from grill once done.

5. Cut the chicken into diagonal pieces. Lay the avocado slices, mango slices and salad greens on the plate and place the chicken pieces on top to serve. Enjoy!

45. Holiday Chicken Salad

Servings: 12

Preparation time: 15 minutes

Cooking time: 15 minutes

Ingredients:

- 4 cups of cooked chicken, cubed
- 1 cup of celery, chopped
- 1 cup of chopped pecans
- Half cup of paleo mayonnaise (preferably homemade)
- Sea salt, to taste
- 1/2 cup of minced green bell pepper
- 1 1/2 cups of dried cranberries (organic and paleo)
- 1 teaspoon paleo seasoning salt
- 2 fresh green onions, chopped
- 1 teaspoon of paprika
- Ground black pepper, to taste

Method of preparation:

1. Combine the Paleo mayonnaise with seasoning salt and paprika.
2. Add all the veggies and fruits. Then, combine the chicken pieces with the mixture at the last.
3. Insert the salad in refrigerator and let chill for 1-2 hours before serving.
4. Serve in lettuce leaves cups or in bell pepper cups or over paleo breads.

46. Creamy Chicken Salad

Servings: 6

Preparation time: 2 hours

Cooking time: 40-45 minutes

Ingredients:

- 2 lbs. (907 grams) of skinless chicken breasts (no bones), halved
- 1 tablespoon of lime juice
- 1 tablespoon of Dijon mustard
- 1/2 cup of light paleo mayonnaise
- 1/2 cup Greek style coconut yogurt
- 1/3 cup of celery, chopped
- 1 tablespoon of paleo coconut vinegar
- 1/3 cup of paleo unsweetened dried cranberries (organic)
- 1 teaspoon of pure raw honey
- 2 oz. (56.699 grams) of smoked almonds
- 1/2 teaspoon of kosher salt
- 6 cups of mixed salad greens
- A pinch of black pepper

Method of preparation:

1. Fill up a Dutch oven two thirds up with water. Bring the water to boil.
2. Wrap up each piece of chicken breast halves with heavy duty plastic wraps and drop in the boiling water.
3. Lower the heat a bit.

4. Let the chicken simmer for 40-45 minutes. Once done, unwrap the chicken breast pieces and shred those. Let cool and transfer to refrigerator to allow chilling for 30-40 minutes.
5. Mix the mayonnaise with shredded chicken, cranberries, celery, almonds and the rest. Chill the salad for 1 hour. Enjoy!

47. Mediterranean Chicken Salad

Servings: 3-4

Preparation time: 10 minutes

Ingredients:

- 1 lb. (458 grams) of roasted chicken (organic and paleo)
- 1 head of butter or romaine lettuce
- 1/2 cup of paleo mayonnaise (preferably homemade)
- 1 whole lemon, juiced
- 4 tablespoons of fresh cilantro, roughly chopped
- 1 whole red onion, diced
- Sea salt
- Black pepper

Method of preparation:

1. Shred the roasted chicken mix it well with rest of the ingredients, except the lettuce leaves.
2. Serve the salad as it is or chilled in the lettuce "boats".

48. Chicken Larb Recipe

Servings: 4

Preparation time: 10 minutes

Cooking time: 10-12 minutes

Ingredients:

- 1 1/2 lbs. (680.388 grams) of ground chicken
- 3/4 cup of homemade chicken stock (paleo)
- 2/3 cup of fresh lime juice
- 2 tablespoons of lemongrass (minced or powdered)
- 1/3 cup of mint leaves
- 1/3 cup of paleo fish sauce
- A few chopped cilantro leaves
- 1 tablespoon of raw paleo honey
- 2 teaspoons of paleo chili-garlic sauce
- Kosher salt, to taste
- 1 cup of green onions, sliced
- 3/4 cup shallots, sliced
- 1 whole head of fresh butter lettuce
- 1 tablespoon of Serrano chili, thinly sliced

Method of preparation:

1. Heat up the chicken stock in a stock pot and drop the ground chicken in it. Simmer the chicken for 6-8 minutes while stirring it occasionally to break the lumps. Add the shallots, lemongrass, green onions and Serrano chilies.

2. In the meantime, combine the honey, fish sauce, lime juice and chili garlic sauce in a bowl and set aside (our salad dressing)
3. Stir and cook the chicken for 4-5 minutes or until the shallots turn translucent.
4. Once cooked, drain the entire liquid from the stock pot and then toss the chicken mixture with the chili garlic sauce mixture.
5. Serve in lettuce leaves boats.

49. *Chipotle Chicken Salad*

Servings: 2-3

Preparation time: 10 minutes

Ingredients:

- 1 lb. (453.592 grams) of cooked chicken, diced
- 1/4 of a white onion (peeled, chopped)
- 4 stalks of celery, finely chopped

For the Paleo mayonnaise (non-vegan):

- 2/3 cup of organic avocado oil
- A pinch of black pepper
- 1 organic egg
- Sea salt
- Fresh lemon juice (1 teaspoon)
- 1/4 teaspoon of organic garlic powder
- 1 teaspoon chipotle adobo sauce (paleo)
- Black pepper, to taste

Method of preparation:

1. To prepare the mayonnaise, blend all the mayonnaise ingredients in a bowl until completely blended and smooth.
2. Mix the chicken with celery and white onions. Add some Paleo mayo and serve. Enjoy!

50. Classic Chicken Salad

Servings: 5-6

Preparation time: 10 minutes

Ingredients:

- 2 lbs. (907 grams) of cooked chicken, cubed or shredded
- 2-3 stalks celery, chopped
- 1 cup of fresh grapes, cut in halves
- 1/3 cup of pecans, chopped (optional)
- 1/2 cup of apple, peeled and chopped (optional)
- 5 teaspoons lemon garlic pepper (paleo)
- 1/2 cup of chopped white or red onion
- 1 cup of paleo mayo (check out the previous recipes)
- 1/2-1 tablespoon of fresh lemon juice
- 2 teaspoons of paleo Trader Joe's 21 Seasoning Salute
- 1 teaspoon of sea salt

Method of preparation:

1. Cube or shred the chicken and add all the fruits, vegetables and nuts to the chicken after chopping and cutting those in the manner as is mentioned.
2. Slowly add the mayonnaise and then add the seasoning, sea salt and pepper. Give a light toss to the salad and serve right away.

51. Chicken with Roasted Asparagus and Bacon Salad

Servings: 2

Preparation time: 10-15 minutes

Cooking time: 10-15 minutes

Ingredients:

- 4 slices of thick cut bacon, paleo
- 6 oz. (200g) of leftover cooked chicken, cut into bite size pieces
- 1 whole ripe avocado, peeled pitted and sliced
- 1/2 cup of asparagus, chopped into 2-3 inch pieces
- 4 cups of baby spinach leaves, chopped
- For the vinaigrette:
- A few tablespoons of olive oil
- 1 teaspoon Dijon mustard
- 2 tablespoons of paleo balsamic vinegar
- 2 teaspoons rosemary, finely chopped
- 1 large clove garlic (peeled and minced)
- 1 tablespoon of thyme, minced
- 1/2 teaspoon of black pepper
- A pinch of Himalayan salt

Method of preparation:

1. Cook the bacon over medium heat in a pan until the bacon slices turn brown and crispy. Once that happens, drain the bacon slices from the pan using a slotted spoon and set aside.

2. Chop the asparagus and dump in the same pan over the bacon drippings. Stir fry the asparagus for 4-5 minutes or until the asparagus gets imbued with the bacon flavors. Turn off the heat once done and set the pan aside.
3. Now dump all the ingredients for the vinaigrette in a small bowl or glass jar and whisk with a metal whisk to get the vinaigrette. The vinaigrette should have a bit emulsified look.
4. Lay the baby spinach leaves over a salad platter and sprinkle the cooked chicken pieces and bacon bits over the spinach. Add the avocado slices as well and then drizzle a little bit of vinaigrette on top to serve immediately.

52. Kiwi-Strawberry Chicken Tender Salad

Servings: 2

Preparation time: 30-40 minutes

Cooking time: 22 minutes

Ingredients:

- 1 lb. (453.592 grams) of chicken cutlets, cut vertically into tenders
- 1 cup of almond flour
- 1 organic egg
- 1½ whole kiwis
- 4 tablespoons of organic raisins
- 1/4th lb. (113 grams) of strawberries
- 3 oz. (85 grams) of fresh baby spinach
- 1 tablespoon of maple syrup, organic and paleo
- 1 whole fresh avocado
- 5 strawberries, sliced
- Sea salt, to taste
- 2 teaspoons of organic honey
- Black pepper, to taste
- Juice of ½ organic lemon
- 1 cup of shredded carrots
- Cucumber, sliced

Method of preparation:

1. Process the 1/4th lb. of strawberries and kiwis in a juicer to extract the juice of these fruits. Mix and combine the maple

syrup thoroughly with the strawberry kiwi juice and set aside.

2. Whisk the egg in another bowl and add 2 tablespoons worth of the strawberry kiwi juice and a dash of sea salt and black pepper to it. Stir to combine.
3. Take the almond flour in another separate bowl.
4. Slice up the chicken cutlets into thin chicken tenders. Take a chicken tender and dunk that in the egg mixture. Transfer the chicken tenders to the almond flour and coat nicely on all sides. Once done, transfer the coated chicken tenders to a greased baking sheet. Repeat the same process with all the remaining chicken tenders.
5. Bake the chicken tenders in a 400 degrees Fahrenheit preheated oven for 20 minutes. Then turn on the broil and broil those for an additional 2 minutes.
6. In the meantime, prepare the salad while the chicken is baking. For that, place half of the fresh baby spinach leaves in a bowl. Dump the avocado in the bowl and add 2 tablespoons worth of the strawberry kiwi juice to the avocado. Mash the avocado with the juices into the spinach.
7. Then add the shredded carrots, 4 sliced strawberries, raisins, lemon juice and a dash of salt and pepper to the salad.
8. Then add the remaining strawberry and cucumbers. Finally top with the baked chicken tenders.
9. Mix the remaining honey with the strawberry kiwi juice and drizzle that over the salad. Enjoy!

53. *Shawarma Chicken Salad with Basil-Lemon Vinaigrette*

Servings: 4

Preparation time: 10 minutes

Cooking time: 13 hours

Ingredients for shawarma:

- 1 lb. (453 grams) of free-range chicken breasts, sliced into 3-inch sized strips
- 3 minced garlic cloves,
- 1 tablespoon of olive oil
- A pinch of ground cumin
- 2 tablespoons of fresh lemon juice
- 1 teaspoon curry powder
- ¾ teaspoon of fine grain sea salt
- ¼ teaspoon of ground coriander

Salad:

- 3.5 oz. (100 grams) of fresh spring greens
- 2 handfuls of fresh basil leaves, torn roughly
- 5oz. (150 grams) of fresh cherry tomatoes cut in halves
- 1 whole avocado, peeled, pitted and sliced

Basil-Lemon Vinaigrette:

- 1 clove of garlic, peeled and smashed

99

- 2 large handfuls of fresh basil leaves
- 5 tablespoons olive oil
- ½ teaspoon of fine grained sea salt
- 2 tablespoons of lemon juice

Method of preparation:

1. Whisk lemon juice, olive oil, curry powder, cumin, garlic, coriander and salt in a bowl to prepare the marinade.
2. Pack the chicken strips into a sealable pouch and add the marinade. Seal and let the chicken sit in the marinade overnight or at least for 20 minutes.
3. When ready to cook, take a skillet and heat up a little amount of olive oil and fry the marinated chicken over medium heat, until the chicken strips attain a golden brown color, for about 6-8 minutes.
4. To prepare the vinaigrette, process the basil, lemon juice, garlic and sea salt in a food processor.
5. Once the mixture turns pasty, start adding the olive oil slowly. Process for a couple of minutes, until you obtain well-combined and smooth vinaigrette.
6. In a bowl, toss the salad green with some salt and pepper and drop the cherry tomatoes, avocado slices, basil and cooked chicken pieces on top. Finally, drizzle the vinaigrette on top and serve. Enjoy!

54. Chicken Salad with Spinach and Strawberries

Servings: 2 - 4

Preparation time: 15-20 minutes

Ingredients:

- 12 oz. (340 grams) of cooked chicken, cubed
- 2 cups of fresh strawberries, sliced
- 8 oz. (227 grams) of fresh baby spinach
- 4 tablespoons of chopped walnuts

Dressing:

- 1 tablespoon of coconut vinegar
- 4 tablespoons of walnut oil
- 1/2 teaspoon of paleo Dijon mustard
- 1 teaspoon of raw honey
- Some pepper
- Sea salt, to taste

Method of preparation:

1. Whisk the honey, walnut oil, Dijon mustard, coconut vinegar, ground black pepper and sea salt in a bowl until the dressing becomes smooth and you get a well combined dressing.

2. Slice the strawberries, chop the walnuts and cut the chicken into small cubes.
3. Combine the spinach with walnuts, strawberries and chicken and drizzle the prepared dressing over the salad.
4. Toss the salad lightly to mix well and serve immediately. Enjoy!

55. Chicken with Charred Tomato and Broccoli Salad

Servings: 6

Preparation time: 20-25 minutes

Cooking time: 10-15 minutes

Ingredients:

- 3 cups of cooked chicken breast, shredded
- 1 1/2 lbs. (680 grams) of medium sized ripe tomatoes
- 1/4th cup of fresh lemon juice
- 3 tablespoons of olive oil
- 4 cups broccoli florets
- A pinch (or more if you like it hot) of chili powder
- 2 teaspoons of extra-virgin olive oil
- 1 teaspoon of sea salt
- Crackled black pepper (1 teaspoon)

Method of preparation:

1. Boil the broccoli florets in a pot of boiling water for about 3-5 minutes Once they get soft, drain the broccoli florets and place the hot florets under some running cold water until the florets cool down.
2. Cut the tomatoes in half horizontally and let the juices and seeds run out. In the meantime, heat up a skillet over high heat. Brush the tops of the halved tomatoes with oil and place those cut side down in the hot pan and let cook for 4-5 minutes or until the tomatoes soften up.

3. Brush the tomatoes again with a teaspoon of olive oil and place back in the pan to let the skin get charred for 1-2 minutes. Once done, remove the tomatoes from the pan.
4. Add some olive oil to the pan and add sea salt, chili powder and ground black pepper. Stir the mixture constantly and cook for 40-45 minutes or until the mixture turns fragrant. Then add in the lemon juice, stir well to combine and then remove from heat.
5. Chop the tomatoes and then toss the tomatoes with shredded chicken and broccoli florets. Drizzle some lemon juice dressing, serve and enjoy!

56. *Chicken Salad with Pecans and Cherries*

Servings: 4

Preparation time: 20-30 minutes

Cooking time: 20-25 minutes

Ingredients:

- 1 1/4 lbs. (567 grams) of chicken breasts, skinless and boneless trimmed
- 1/3 cup of paleo mayonnaise
- 1/2 cup of celery (sliced)
- 1/2 cup of pecans, slightly toasted and chopped
- 1 head of butterhead lettuce, chopped
- 1/2 cup of dried cherries
- 1/3 cup of coconut yogurt
- A pinch of sea salt
- 1 tablespoon raw honey mustard

Method of preparation:

1. Fill up a pot with some water and add 1/4th teaspoon of sea salt to it. Bring the water in the pot to boil and then drop the chicken breasts in it. Once the chicken breasts start boiling, reduce the heat and cover the pot with a lid. Let the chicken simmer for 20-25 minutes or until the time those are cooked through, tender and are no longer pink. Once done, drain the water and let the chicken cool down.
2. Mix up the paleo mayonnaise with coconut yoghurt, black pepper, mustard and remaining salt in a bowl.

3. Cut up the chicken breasts into small pieces once the chicken breasts cool down.
4. Toss the chicken pieces with cherries, celery and pecans. Add the prepared mayonnaise dressing and mix well.
5. Serve the salad over the lettuce. Enjoy!

57. Chopped Chicken Greek Salad

Servings: 4

Preparation time: 15-20 minutes

Ingredients:

- 12 oz. (340 grams) of cooked chicken, chopped
- 6 cups of chopped romaine lettuce
- 1/2 cup of crumbled paleo feta cheese***
- Optional: 1/3 cup of paleo vinegar (or red wine- allowed on Paleo)
- 2 medium sized tomatoes, chopped
- 2 tablespoons of olive oil (extra-virgin)
- 1/2 cup of sliced ripe black olives
- 1 tablespoon of fresh dill, chopped
- 1 medium sized cucumber, peeled, chopped
- 1 teaspoon of garlic powder
- 1/4 teaspoon Himalaya salt
- 1 onion, chopped
- A pinch of freshly ground pepper

***To make Paleo Cashew Feta Style Cheese, simply blend the following ingredients: 1 cup of raw cashews previously soaked in water for at least a few hours (I leave it to soak overnight and I use alkaline water), about ¼ cup of almond milk or coconut milk, 1 tablespoon of lime juice, ¼ cup of nutritional yeast, 1 clove of garlic and a bit of Himalaya salt to taste. Transfer into little cubes (like for ice making) and store in a fridge for a few hours.

Method of preparation:

1. Toss the olives, romaine lettuce, paleo feta cheese, cucumber, onions, tomatoes and chicken cubes in a bowl.
2. Whisk some olive oil, red wine, dill, ground black pepper and sea salt in a bowl.
3. Drizzle the dressing over the salad and toss again before serving. Enjoy!

58. Orange Five Spice Chicken Salad

Servings: 4

Preparation time: 15-20 minutes

Cooking time: 15-17 minutes

Ingredients:

- 1 lb. (458 grams) of skinless and boneless chicken breasts, trimmed
- 3 whole fresh oranges
- 1 tablespoon of Dijon mustard
- 12 cups of mixed Asian greens
- 3 tablespoons of coconut vinegar
- 6 teaspoons of extra-virgin olive oil
- 1 red bell pepper, with no seeds
- 1 teaspoon of five-spice powder, organic
- 1/2 cup of slivered red onion
- 1 teaspoon of kosher salt, divided
- A pinch of freshly ground black pepper

Method of preparation:

1. In a bowl, combine the five spice powder, some olive oil, salt and black pepper so as to prepare a spice rub.
2. Coat the chicken breast pieces with the spice rub.
3. In a skillet, heat up a bit of olive oil and brown the spiced chicken pieces. Once browned on one side, flip the chicken pieces and pop the skillet into a 450 degrees Fahrenheit oven.
4. Roast the chicken in the oven for about 10 minutes.

5. Once cooked, set aside to cool down.
6. Finally, shred the chicken and toss with the salad ingredients. Enjoy!

SECTION 4 MORE AMAZING PALEO SALADS

59. Red Potato Honey Mustard Salad

Servings: 4

Preparation time: 15 minutes

Cooking time: 15 minutes

Ingredients:

- 3 lbs. (1.36 kg) of red potatoes, cut into 1inch sized pieces
- 3 slices of thick cut bacon
- 3 tablespoons of homemade paleo mayonnaise
- 3 tablespoons of organic honey
- 2 medium sized onions, peeled and chopped
- 4 tablespoons of Dijon mustard
- 3 tablespoons of organic coconut vinegar
- 1/3rd cup of parsley
- 1 teaspoon of black pepper
- ½ teaspoon of sea salt

Method of preparation:

1. Boil the red potatoes in a pot of water and once boiling, lower the heat to simmer until the potatoes are cooked through and can be pierced with a knife or fork. Drain and set aside.

2. In the meantime, cook the bacon slices until all the fat is released. Add the onion slices and sauté those in bacon fat until caramelized.
3. Prepare the honey dressing by mixing mayonnaise, honey, Dijon mustard and coconut vinegar.
4. Toss the potatoes with sea salt, bacon and onion mixture, parsley and black pepper. Serve immediately or after chilling. Enjoy!

60 Duck with Sprout and Brussels Salad

Servings: 2

Preparation time: 15 minutes

Cooking time: 30-35 minutes

Ingredients:

- 2 pieces of duck breasts, skin on
- 2 whole clementine oranges
- 4 cups of Brussels sprouts, quartered
- 1/3 cup of organic dried cranberries
- 2 fennel stalks, finely chopped
- 1 tablespoon of coconut oil
- Coconut aminos (2 tablespoons)
- 2 teaspoons of black pepper
- 2 teaspoons of sea salt

Method of preparation:

1. Set up a temperature preheating of 375 degrees Fahrenheit on an oven. Scour the skin of duck breasts lightly on both sides and then sprinkle a dash of ground black pepper and sea salt on both the sides to season.
2. Transfer duck breasts to a skillet and cover the skillet with a parchment paper. Cook the duck for about 15 minutes and then flip.
3. Drain half of the coconut oil from skillet and transfer the skillet to the preheated oven.
4. Allow the duck to bake for 10-15 minutes.
5. While the duck is baking in the oven, heat up reserved coconut oil and fry the Brussels sprouts, cranberries and

fennel in it. Stir and cook for a minute and then add the coconut aminos. Stir to combine well. Then cook for 7-8 minutes or until the sprouts turn tender.

6. Slice the duck breasts and serve over cooked sprouts mixture. Drizzle clementine juice on top to serve.

61. Paleo Turkey Salad

Servings: 2

Preparation time: 10 minutes

Ingredients:

- 0.55 oz. (250g) of cooked turkey, cubed
- 4 tablespoons of chopped walnuts
- 1 whole avocado, peeled and diced
- 1/2 cup of fresh cranberries, halved
- 3 whole clementine oranges, sections halved
- 4 tablespoons of raw raisins
- 1 large endive, julienned
- 1/4 cup of fresh parsley
- 1/2 cup raw broccoli florets, chopped finely

Method of preparation:

1. Peel, cut and chop the vegetables and fruits as is required and mentioned in ingredients list.
2. Combine all of the added ingredients using a large salad bowl. Toss the salad and serve with dressing of choice or refrigerate for later use. Enjoy!

62. *Paleo Taco Salad*

Servings: 5-6

Preparation time: 15 minutes

Cooking time: 10 minutes

Ingredients:

- 2 lbs. (907 grams) of organic ground beef, cooked (leftovers will work well)
- 1 lb. (453.592 grams) of cooked bacon bits (organic)
- 1 large sized head of lettuce
- 3 whole avocados, peeled and pitted
- Paleo chimichurri (optional)
- Olive oil
- 2 whole fresh tomatoes
- 2 fresh red apples
- Apple cider vinegar (optional)
- Ground black pepper
- Sea salt

Method of preparation:

1. Season the meat with salt, olive oil and black pepper as required. Cool down if necessary.
2. Mix the cooled browned ground beef with the rest of the ingredients. Enjoy!

63. *Salade Lyonnaise*

Servings: 2

Preparations time: 15-20 minutes

Cooking time: 15-17 minutes

Ingredients:

- 1/4th lb. (113.398 grams) of thick-cut bacon
- 4 cups of fresh salad greens
- 2 poached eggs, organic
- 2 tablespoons of minced shallot
- 1 teaspoon of coconut vinegar
- Black pepper, to taste
- 1 tablespoon of organic ground mustard
- Salt, to taste

Method of preparation:

1. Bring a pot of water to boil and heat up another pan. Once water steams up, drop the eggs one by one at a time in it to poach those.
2. Fry the bacon bits for 10-12 minutes or unless those are browned and crispy. Season as required. Drain bacon bits in paper towels and set aside.
3. Cook the shallots lightly in the bacon fat and then add the mustard and vinegar. Stir nicely to mix. Then, cook for a couple of minutes.
4. Toss the salad greens with shallot mustard mixture and then serve with the bacon bits and pierced poached eggs on top. Enjoy!

64. Paleo Indonesian Shrimp Salad

Servings: 3-4

Preparation time: 10-15 minutes

Ingredients:

- 1 lb. (453.592 grams) of cooked shrimp, halved vertically
- 1.5 tablespoons of paleo fish sauce
- 3 whole fresh carrots, roughly shredded
- 6 tablespoons of raw almond butter (paleo)
- 1 whole seedless cucumber, julienned
- 6 tablespoons of raw unsweetened coconut milk (organic and paleo)
- 1 yellow or red bell pepper, seeded and sliced very thinly
- 1 teaspoon of paleo home-made sriracha sauce
- Raw organic cashews nuts, for garnishing
- 2 teaspoons of organic palm sugar (optional)
- 1 tablespoon of chopped scallions, for garnishing
- Juice of 1/2 lime
- 2 romaine lettuce hearts, coarsely shredded
- Lime wedges, for garnishing

Here's how to make your own sriracha sauce, all you need is a blender and:

- 1 cup of red jalapeño peppers, chopped
- 6 garlic cloves, peeled
- ¼ cup apple cider vinegar (this is not strictly Paleo, but many modern Paleo followers accept it as "legal" as it has many health benefits)
- 2 tablespoons organic honey
- 2 tablespoons Paleo-friendly fish sauce

- 1 teaspoon Himalaya salt
- 4 tablespoons tomato sauce (home-made)

Method: blend, cool down in a fridge and enjoy. This recipe makes about 1 cup of sriracha sauce.

Method of preparation:

1. Chop all the vegetables and shrimps as is mentioned in the ingredients list. Toss the vegetables in a salad bowl.
2. Now combine the palm sugar, almond butter, lime juice, sriracha sauce, coconut milk and fish sauce in a food processor. Process until the palm sugar breaks and you get a smooth salad dressing.
3. Add the cooked shrimps to the vegetables mixture after slitting those halfway lengthwise through the middle.
4. Add the palm sugar salad dressing to the shrimps and vegetables salad and mix well. Garnish with raw cashews, lime wedges and chopped scallions before serving.

65. Paleo Seafood Salad

Servings: 3-4

Preparation time: 12 hours

Ingredients:

- 8 oz. (226.796 grams) of cooked baby shrimps, shelled and chopped
- 2/3 cup of homemade paleo mayonnaise
- 8 oz. (226.796 grams) of sweet crab meat
- 2/3 cup of chopped celery
- 1/2 teaspoon of organic celery salt
- 1 cup of finely chopped white onion
- 1/2 teaspoon of garlic powder
- 1 tablespoon of hot sauce (you can use the one from the previous recipe)
- 2 tablespoons Dijon mustard
- 1/4 teaspoon of onion powder

Method of preparation:

1. Chop the celery and the white onion as required. Add the chopped shrimps and crab meat.
2. Add the rest of the ingredients and toss together to coat.
3. Transfer the salad to an air right refrigerator compatible container and serve the salad chilled within a few hours (or the next day). Perfect for those who like to have their food prepared in advance!

66. Bacon Brussels Salad

Servings: 10

Preparation time: 40 minutes

Ingredients:

- 6 whole slices of organic cooked bacon, chopped or crumbled
- 1 cup of grated paleo home-made cashew parmesan cheese*
- 1 whole orange
- 1 cup of almonds
- 1/2 cup olive oil
- 1 whole lemon
- 4 dozens of Brussels sprouts
- 1 large sized shallot, finely chopped
- A dash of black pepper
- Sea salt, to taste

*Vegan Paleo Parmesan Cheese is super easy to make. All you need is to blend: 1 cup of raw cashews with ¼ cup of nutritional yeast and a bit of Himalaya salt. No excuses now. Cutting out dairy is easy if you prepare yourself with the right ingredients.

Method of preparation:

1. Place the shallots in a bowl. Add the lemon and orange juice as well as olive oil while whisking the mixture constantly to prepare an emulsion. Transfer the emulsion to refrigerator and let sit for a few hours.

2. Cook the bacon slices in a skillet until crispy and all done. Crumble or cut the bacon slices into small bite sized pieces. Drain and set aside.
3. Shave the Brussels sprouts and add the crumbled Paleo cheese and bacon pieces to the sprouts.
4. Process the almonds in a food processor.
5. Add the crumbled almonds and olive oil emulsion to the sprouts salad and toss well to combine. Enjoy!

67.Crabmeat Spinach Salad

Servings: 4

Preparation time: 10 minutes

Ingredients:

- 1/2 lb. (680.389 grams) of cooked crabmeat
- 2 bunch of spinach leaves, rinsed
- 2 large sized tomatoes, thinly sliced
- 2 pieces of hardboiled eggs, thinly sliced
- 1 Maui sweet onion, sliced thinly

Ingredients for salad dressing:

- 1 cup of fresh tomato puree
- 1 teaspoon of cayenne pepper
- 3 tablespoons of dry mustard powder (organic)
- 2 cup of flaxseed oil
- 1 tablespoon of ground black pepper
- 1 cup of freshly extracted lemon juice
- 1 large clove of garlic, peeled and minced
- 1 cup of paleo burgundy wine
- 1 tablespoon of black pepper

Method of preparation:

1. Blend the salad dressing ingredients and set aside.
2. Mix the crabmeat with spinach leaves pieces, sliced sweet onion, egg slices and tomato slices.

3. Add the required amount of salad dressing to the salad and toss lightly to coat and serve immediately. Enjoy!

68.Seared Scallops Salad with Arugula

Servings: 4

Preparation time: 15 minutes

Cooking time: 50-55 minutes

Ingredients:

- 1 lb. (453.592 grams) of sea scallops
- 2 garlic cloves, peeled and minced (you can also use garlic powder)
- 3oz. of baby arugula, rinsed and chopped
- 1 teaspoon of fresh lemon zest
- 4 tablespoons of olive oil
- 2 tablespoons of fresh lemon juice
- 1/4 teaspoon of ground black pepper
- 2 teaspoons of kosher salt

Method of preparation:

1. To prepare the salad dressing, combine the minced garlic with salt, black pepper and lemon zest with lemon juice. Whisk to combine well. Now slowly and steadily add the olive oil while whisking continuously to form the dressing. Set aside the dressing to let the flavors marry for 15 minutes.
2. Toss the salad dressing with arugula. Set aside.
3. Rinse and dry the scallops. Season those with salt and pepper.
4. Heat up oil in a large skillet and place the seasoned scallops in it once the oil turns hot. Sear the scallops for 3-4 minutes

or until golden browned. Flip the scallops and sear the other side for 1-2 minutes. Drain and set the scallops aside.

5. Serve the seared scallops over the arugula salad. Enjoy!

69. Yummy Sesame Beef Salad

Servings: 4

Preparation time: 20-25 minutes

Cooking time: 15-20 minutes

Ingredients:

- 2lbs. (907 grams) of ground beef or bison
- 2 tablespoons of paleo Worcestershire sauce
- 1 bunch of scallions, sliced
- 2 garlic cloves, peeled and minced
- 1 carrot, peeled and grated
- 1/2 head of red cabbage, sliced thinly into ribbons
- 2 tablespoons of coconut aminos
- 1/2 cup of fresh cilantro leaves, chopped
- 8 oz. (226.8 grams) of fresh mixed greens of your choice
- A dash of cayenne pepper
- 1 tablespoons of sesame oil
- 2 tablespoons of sesame seeds
- Kosher salt, to taste
- 1 whole lime, juiced
- Some ground black pepper, to taste

Method of preparation:

1. Toast the sesame seeds until golden. Remove from hot pan and set aside to prevent the seeds from scorching.
2. Dump the ground beef in the same pan and cook until beef is browned and no longer in lumps. Add the garlic and cayenne pepper to the beef and stir to combine nicely.
3. Finally add the coconut aminos, salt, black pepper, lime juice and Worcestershire sauce to the beef. Give a nice stir

to mix everything up thoroughly. Once done, turn off the heat and remove from pan.

4. Chop and slice the cabbage, carrot, and scallions. Add cilantro leaves. Toss the vegetables and mixed greens with sesame oil.

5. Top the vegetables and mixed greens with the browned beef and serve.

70.Sirloin Salad with Balsamic Vinaigrette

Servings: 2-4

Preparation time: 15 minutes

Cooking time: 5 minutes

Ingredients:

- 1/2 cup of bacon bits, fried
- 1/2 lb. (226.8 grams) of grass-fed sirloin, cooked and sliced
- 1/2 cup of fresh cherry tomatoes, halved
- 1/2 cup of almonds
- 1/2 cup of red onion rings
- 1/2 cup of dried cranberries
- Dressing:
- 4 tablespoons of coconut vinegar
- 3/4 cup of olive oil (extra virgin)
- 2 garlic cloves, peeled
- Salt, to taste
- Black pepper, to taste

Method of preparation:

1. Arrange all the salad ingredients side by side in a salad platter and place the cooked sirloin at the middle.
2. To prepare the dressing, process everything together (except for the oil) until a smooth dressing is formed. Add the extra virgin olive oil at the end while still processing the mixture.
3. Once everything is ready, serve the dressing beside the salad.

71. *Avocado BLT Egg Salad*

Servings: 3-4

Preparation time: 10 minutes

Cooking time: 10 minutes

Ingredients:

- 4 strips of bacon, cooked until crispy
- 1 whole avocado
- 1/2 cup of fresh scallions, chopped
- 6 hard-boiled eggs
- 2 teaspoon of ground garlic
- 1/2 teaspoon of Himalayan sea salt, more to taste
- 3/4th cup of grape tomatoes cut in halves

Method of preparation:

1. Combine the hard boiled eggs with avocado, sea salt and ground garlic. Do not mash the eggs completely.
2. Finally add the rest of the ingredients to the eggs mixture and serve immediately.

72. *Bacon Fennel Salad with Grilled Peaches*

Servings: 4-6

Preparation time: 30-40 minutes

Cooking time: 20-25 minutes

Ingredients:

- 1 cup of chopped fennel bulb
- 4 slices of bacon, cooked and chopped into small bits
- 1 tablespoon of melted coconut oil
- 3-4 ripe peaches
- 1 tablespoon of coconut oil
- 1/2 lb. (226.8 grams) of mixed salad greens
- A pinch of celtic sea salt

For the dressing:

- 4 whole dried dates, pitted
- 5 tablespoons of olive oil
- 1 strip of cooked bacon
- 2 tablespoons of bacon fat
- 2 tablespoons of coconut vinegar
- 1/4 teaspoon of celtic sea salt

Method of preparation:

1. Heat up 1 tablespoon of coconut oil in a skillet and drop the chopped fennel in it. Sauté the fennel until cooked and aromatic, for about 4-5 minutes. Once done, drain the fennel and set aside.
2. To prepare the grilled peaches, cut those in half and pit the halves. Grease the cut side of the peach slices with remaining coconut oil and place on the grill. Grill the peaches lid-on over medium heat for 12-15 minutes or until the peaches turn tender and start falling apart.
3. To prepare the salad dressing, blend all the ingredients required until everything is processed and the dressing is smooth and lump free.
4. Toss the salad greens along with the salad dressing. Add the cooked bacon, grilled peach halves and fennel to the salad. Serve right away.

73. Back Ribs Cherry Cabbage Slaw

Servings: 4-6

Preparation time: 20-25 minutes

Cooking time:1 hour 30 minutes

Ingredients:

- 1 entire rack of pork ribs, cut in half crosswise

Spice rub:

- 1 tablespoon of ground ancho chiles
- 1 teaspoon of celery seed
- 1 tablespoon of dried thyme
- 1 teaspoon of ground mustard
- 1 tablespoon of garlic powder
- 1 teaspoon of cayenne
- 1 tablespoon of onion powder
- 1 teaspoon dried rosemary
- 1 tablespoon of smoked paprika
- 1 teaspoon of sea salt

Cherry cabbage slaw:

- 2 medium sized carrots, shredded
- 1/2 of a cabbage head, cored and thinly sliced

- Juice of 2 limes
- Zest of 2 limes
- 2 cups of fresh cherries, pitted and halved
- 1/2 of a red onion, peeled and thinly sliced
- 4 tablespoons of olive oil
- Sea salt
- Black pepper

Method of preparation:

1. Prepare spice rub by mixing all the ground spices together. Rub the salad rub over the pork ribs and transfer the ribs to a baking dish (add ¼ cup water).
2. Bake the pork ribs in a 325 degrees Fahrenheit (or: 160 Celsius) oven for 80-85 minutes. Once done, remove the pork from oven and set aside.
3. Set the grill to medium high and grill the ribs for 10-12 minutes or until the ribs are crispy.
4. Finally, toss the cabbage, cherries, onion and carrots with olive oil, lime zest, lime juice, sea salt and black pepper to prepare the slaw.
5. Serve the grilled ribs alongside the slaw.

SECTION 5 FRUIT SALADS

74. Pink Grapefruit with Avocado Salad

Servings: 4

Preparation time: 10 minutes

Ingredients:

- 2 whole avocados
- 1 tablespoon of extra virgin olive oil
- A pinch of sea salt
- 2 grapefruits
- 1 tablespoon of coconut vinegar

Method of preparation:

1. Slice the avocados in halves. Remove the pits and cut the avocado flesh into small cubes or slices.
2. Segment the grapefruits and add the pieces to the avocado chunks.
3. Whisk the coconut vinegar with some olive oil. Add sea salt and mix well. Pour over the salad and serve. Enjoy! This salad is extremely alkaline and will help you balance your pH.

75. *Waldorf-ish Salad*

Servings: 4-5

Preparation time: 10 minutes

Cooking time: 5 minutes

Ingredients:

- 3 medium sized organic red apples, cored and diced
- 1 1/2 teaspoon of organic maple syrup
- 3 stalks of celery, sliced on the bias
- 4 tablespoons of pecans
- 1 teaspoon of coconut butter
- 1 tablespoon of paleo apple cider vinegar
- 2 tablespoons of coconut cream
- A pinch of cayenne pepper
- Sea salt
- Ground black pepper, to taste

Method of preparation:

1. Melt the coco butter and add 1 teaspoon of maple syrup to it (use a small frying-pan). Drop the pecans in the mixture and stir energetically.
2. Cook for 3-4 minutes or until the pecans turn golden brown. Once done, drain and allow to cool down.
3. Slice and dice the celery and the apples. Place in a salad bowl.
4. Combine the remaining maple syrup with coconut cream, apple cider vinegar, cayenne pepper, salt and ground black pepper.
5. Drizzle salad dressing on top of salad, add the pecans and toss with salad. Enjoy!

76. Simple Pear and Walnut Salad

Servings: 4

Preparation time: 8-10 minutes

Ingredients:

- 1/2 cup of dried cherries
- 3/4th cup of walnuts, organic
- 2 ripe pears
- 5 cups of salad greens
- 2 tablespoons of coconut milk
- Juice of 2 lemons

Method of preparation:

1. Cut the pears into bite sized pieces and transfer to a salad bowl.
2. Add the walnuts, salad greens and dried cherries to the pears and toss nicely.
3. Serve the salad with coconut milk and lemon sauce or any other salad dressings of choice. Enjoy!

77. *Winter Fruit Salad*

Servings: 4

Preparation time: 10-15 minutes

Ingredients:

- 100 grams (3.5 oz.) of fresh rocket leaves
- 1/2 fresh lemon
- 2 blood oranges, peeled and halved horizontally
- 1.05 oz. (30 grams) of paleo cashew cheese (mentioned in previous recipes)
- 1 whole pomegranate, seeded
- A few small sprigs of mint, leaves separated
- Some olive oil

Method of preparation:

1. Rinse the rocket leaves. Drain and set aside. Peel and slice the oranges and then seed the pomegranate.
2. To prepare the dressing, whisk together lemon juice, salt and olive oil.
3. Toss the orange pieces and rocket leaves with the dressing and then transfer to serving plates.
4. Drop the pomegranate seeds and sprinkle over some paleo cheese on top and serve. Enjoy!

78. Papaya Avocado Slaw

Servings: 3-4

Preparation time: 10-15 minutes

Ingredients:

- 10 oz. (283.495 grams) of organic broccoli slaw
- 2 tablespoons of lemon juice
- 1 cup of ripe papaya, cubed
- 2 tablespoons of finely chopped fresh cilantro
- 1/2 avocado, peeled and chopped
- 1/2 tablespoon of paleo balsamic vinegar (not really Paleo, but accepted by many Paleo gurus due to its numerous health benefits)

Method of preparation:

1. Cut the papaya, avocado and chop the cilantro.
2. Mix all the ingredients together in a salad bowl. Serve and enjoy.

79. Grapes and Walnuts Salad

Servings: 8

Preparation time: 5 minutes

Ingredients:

- 2 lbs. (907 grams) of fresh grapes
- 1 cup raw walnut halves
- 2 tablespoons of olive oil
- 3 big avocados, peeled, pitted and diced
- 2 tablespoons of paleo red wine vinegar

Method of preparation:

1. Dump the grapes and the walnut in a large salad bowl. Add avocado pieces on top and toss the salad with some red wine vinegar and olive oil.
2. Refrigerate to chill and serve.

80. Strawberry with Prosciutto Salad

Servings: 2

Preparation time: 10 minutes

Cooking time: 5 minutes

Ingredients:

- 4 cups baby spinach
- 2 oz. (56.7 grams) of smoked almonds
- 2 cups sliced strawberries
- 2 oz. (56.7 grams) of crumbled paleo cheese (use the vegan cashew nut cheese recipe mentioned previously)
- 4 thin slices of prosciutto
- 4 tablespoons of paleo organic balsamic dressing

Method of preparation:

1. Broil the prosciutto slices on high for 5 minutes or until crispy. Cool down.
2. Slice the strawberries and transfer to a bowl. Add the spinach leaves to the strawberry slices.
3. Crumble the paleo cheese and prosciutto slices on top. Drizzle balsamic dressing on top and serve. Enjoy!

81. Pear Apple and Spinach Salad

Servings: 4

Preparation time: 10 minutes

Ingredients:

- 2 medium sized pears, peeled, cored and thinly sliced
- 6 cups of fresh baby spinach
- 1 cup of dried cranberries
- 2 medium sized apples, peeled, cored and sliced thinly
- 1/3 cup of olive oil
- 1 tablespoons of lemon juice
- Some Paleo mustard to taste
- A dash of ground black pepper
- 4 tablespoons of paleo apple cider vinegar
- 1 tablespoon of raw honey
- A dash of sea salt

Method of preparation:

1. Peel, core and slice the apples and pears as mentioned. Pour enough water over the fruit slices, so as to cover the fruits entirely up to the top with water. Place a small sized plate over the fruit slices, so as to make them remain submerged in the water.
2. Prepare the salad dressing by whisking apple cider vinegar with some olive oil, and honey. Add mustard, sea salt, lemon juice and pepper and whisk until there are no clumps in the mixture.

3. Combine the spinach and cranberries in a separate bowl. Drain the fruits and add those to the spinach and cranberries mixture.
4. Drizzle the salad dressing on top and serve. Enjoy!

82. *Lemon Refreshing Fruit Salad*

Servings: 4

Preparation time: 20 minutes

Ingredients:

- 2 large sized Fuji or Gala apples, peeled, cored and cubed
- 2 large sized navel oranges, peeled and sliced
- 2 large sized mangoes, peeled and cubed
- 2 teaspoons of finely grated fresh ginger
- 2 large sized red Bartlett pears
- 2 tablespoons of organic honey
- 1 pineapple, peeled, cored and cubed
- 4 tablespoons of fresh lemon juice

Method of preparation:

1. Peel and cut the apples, mangoes, pears, oranges and pineapple into small bite sized pieces or cubes.
2. Mix the lemon juice, grated ginger and honey in a bowl to prepare the salad dressing.
3. Pour the salad dressing over the salad and toss to finish the preparation.

83. Peach Nectarine and Strawberry Salad with Honey Lime Basil Syrup

Servings: 6

Preparation time: 10 minutes

Ingredients:

- 6 large sized strawberries
- 1 whole lime
- 1 tablespoon lime zest
- 3 white peaches
- 1 tablespoon of honey
- 3 large nectarines
- 1 tablespoon chopped fresh basil

Method of preparation:

1. Quarter the strawberries and cut the nectarines and peaches into bite sized pieces.
2. Prepare the syrup by mixing honey with basil and lime juice.
3. Mix all the fruits in a salad bowl. Sprinkle over some lemon zest and syrup to the salad.
4. Toss to mix and serve right away. Enjoy!

84. Strawberry Caprese Salad

Servings: 1

Preparation time: 5 minutes

Ingredients:

- 10 whole strawberries
- Extra virgin olive oil
- 3.5oz (100 g) of paleo vegan mozzarella cheese***
- Crushed black pepper (to taste)
- 15 fresh organic basil leaves

Method of preparation:

1. Quarter the strawberries and add the paleo mozzarella cheese.
2. Add the basil leaves and season the salad with black pepper.
3. Drizzle desired amount of olive oil over the salad. Toss the salad and serve to enjoy.

***Here's what you need to make Paleo mozzarella cheese:

- 1/2 cup of thick coconut milk
- 1 cup coconut butter, half-melted
- Half cup of melted coconut oil
- Nutritional yeast (4 tablespoons)
- A pinch of Himalaya salt
- Juice of 2 lemons
- 1 teaspoon of garlic powder (yummy!)
- Half cup of melted coconut oil

1. Blend all the ingredients adding melted coconut oil last. Blend again until 100% smooth.
2. Pour into a freezer-safe container and freeze for about 1 hour.
3. Serve with salads, enjoy!

85. Nutty Fruity Salad

Servings: 2

Preparation time: 10-12 minutes

Ingredients:

- 1 whole apple, cubed
- 1 whole banana, peeled and sliced
- 1 whole orange, cut into segments
- 1/4 of a pineapple, cut into cubes
- A handful of sunflower seeds
- 6-7 fresh strawberries, halved
- A handful of almonds
- A handful of organic pumpkin seeds

Method of preparation:

1. Peel and slice the banana, cut the apples and pineapples into cubes and segment the orange.
2. Transfer the chopped fruits to a salad bowl.
3. Add the nuts and seeds to the fruits and toss lightly to mix up. Serve immediately.

86. Simple Fruit Salad

Servings: 10

Preparation time: 30-40 minutes

Ingredients:

- 1 whole ripe papaya
- 8-10 lychees, pitted
- 1/2 watermelon, seeded and cut into cubes
- 3 whole mangoes, pitted and cubed
- 5 fresh kiwis, sliced
- 6 apricots, sliced
- 3-4 ripe bananas, sliced
- 2 teaspoons of paleo vanilla extract
- 2 teaspoons cinnamon powder

Method of preparation:

1. Dump all the fruit slices in a large sized salad bowl.
2. Drizzle the vanilla extract and add a dash of cinnamon powder to the salad. Toss the salad slightly and serve fresh.

87. Simple Avocado Alkaline Salad

Servings: 4

Preparation time: 10-15 minutes

Ingredients:

- 2 ripe avocados, mashed or cubed
- ½ of a red onion, peeled and chopped
- 1 whole ripe mango, cubed
- 1 teaspoon of fresh lime juice
- 1 garlic clove, peeled and minced
- ½ red onion, chopped
- A cup of cherry tomatoes, halved
- 1 whole jalapeño, deseeded and minced
- Fresh greens
- 1 Thai red chili, deseeded and minced (optional)
- A dash of avocado oil
- Sea salt, to taste

Method of preparation:

1. Cut and chop the vegetables and fruits. Mix everything up in a salad bowl and serve right away. Enjoy!

BONUS: SECTION 6 PALEO SALAD SAUCES AND CONDIMENTS

Aside from a few condiments and non-dairy Paleo solutions that I have mentioned in this book, I would love to introduce you to my favorite Paleo salad dressings and condiments. Spice up your salads and enjoy variety! Enjoy the creative Paleo ride and design a healthy lifestyle for you and your family.

88 Paleo Tahini Salad Dressing

Servings: 1/4th cup

Preparation time: 5 minutes

Ingredients:

- 2-3 tablespoons of Tahini (sesame seed butter)
- Some organic apple cider vinegar, to taste
- 1 whole lemon, juiced
- Ground black pepper, to taste
- 2 cloves of garlic
- Sea salt, to taste

Method of preparation:

1. Blend all the ingredients until well combined and smooth.
2. Add more water or apple cider vinegar to loosen out dressing, if required.

89. Orange Poppy Dressing

Servings: 2-3

Preparation time: 5-7 minutes

Ingredients:

- 1 tablespoons of paleo Dijon mustard
- 1 orange, juiced
- 1 tablespoon of poppy seeds
- Zest of 1 orange
- 1 whole garlic clove, smashed
- 1 teaspoon of paleo white wine vinegar
- 4 tablespoons of paleo mayonnaise
- 1/4th teaspoon of ground white pepper
- 1/4th teaspoon of Himalayan salt

Method of preparation:

1. Blend all the ingredients until you achieve smooth salad dressing.
2. Toss and serve with a yummy Paleo salad of your choice!

90. Chive and Hemp Oil Salad Dressing

Servings: 1 cup

Preparation time: 5 minutes

Ingredients:

- 1 tablespoon of hemp oil
- 1/2 teaspoon of raw honey
- 1 teaspoon of paleo red wine vinegar
- 1 tablespoon of finely chopped chives
- 1 clove fresh garlic, minced
- 1 tablespoon of extra virgin olive oil

Method of preparation:

1. Combine the red wine vinegar, extra virgin olive oil, hemp oil, chopped chives, honey and minced garlic in a bowl.
2. Whisk the mixture until everything is well combined and you get a smooth salad dressing. Serve with a yummy Paleo salad of your choice!

91. Maple Mustard Dressing

Servings: 4

Preparation time: 4-5 minutes

Ingredients:

- 2 teaspoons of organic maple syrup
- 1 tablespoon light olive oil
- Some black pepper to taste
- 2 tablespoons of organic Dijon mustard

Method of preparation:

1. Take the maple syrup in a small bowl and add Dijon mustard, olive oil and ground black pepper to the maple syrup.
2. Whisk the mixture in the bowl to prepare the salad dressing.
3. Serve with a yummy Paleo salad of your choice!

92. *Carrot Ginger Salad Dressing*

Servings: 6

Preparation time: 6-8 minutes

Ingredients:

- ½ lb. (226.8 grams) of peeled and chopped carrots,
- 4 tablespoons of paleo apple cider vinegar
- 1 tablespoon of coconut aminos
- ¼ cup of fresh ginger, peeled and chopped
- ½ cup olive oil
- 1 chopped onion (small)
- 1/8 teaspoon of sea salt
- 1 tablespoon of sesame oil

Method of preparation:

1. Peel and coarsely chop the carrots. Dump the carrots in food processor and process until the carrots are nicely processed and turn into a paste.
2. Add the coconut aminos, sesame oil, chopped onions, ginger, vinegar and sea salt to the carrots. Process again until the dressing is loosened a bit. Then add some olive oil to it. Process well to combine and serve with a yummy Paleo salad of your choice!

93. *Creamy Citrus Almond Dressing*

Servings: 1

Preparation time: 5 minutes

Ingredients:

- 1 tablespoon of fresh orange juice
- 1 teaspoon of organic almond butter
- Salt, to taste
- 1 tablespoon of avocado oil
- Black pepper, to taste
- 1/4 teaspoon of minced garlic

Method of preparation:

1. Peel and mince the garlic cloves.
2. Blend in a blender. Serve with a yummy Paleo salad of your choice.

94. Tomato Cilantro Dressing

Servings: 4

Preparation time: 5-7 minutes

Ingredients:

- 1 tomato
- 1/4 cup of olive oil
- 2 cloves of garlic, peeled
- 1/2 small red onion
- A handful of fresh cilantro
- 2 green onions
- Sea salt, to taste
- Black pepper, to taste

Method of preparation:

1. Rinse all the vegetables and set aside.
2. Blend all the veggies until everything is fairly nicely processed.
3. Do not make the dressing too smooth. Serve with a yummy Paleo salad of your choice!

95. *Catalina Dressing*

Servings: 1 cup

Preparation time: 5 minutes

Ingredients:

- 2 tablespoons of fresh tomato paste
- ½ cup of olive oil
- 1 teaspoon of Paleo mustard
- 4 tablespoons of raw apple cider vinegar
- Half teaspoon of paprika
- 1 tablespoon of raw honey
- 1teaspoon of onion granules
- 1/2 teaspoon garlic granules
- 1/4 teaspoon of chili powder
- A pinch of black pepper

Method of preparation:

1. Combine all the ingredients and whisk well.
2. Once done, store the salad dressing in a container or jar and serve with any salad of choice.

BONUS Alkaline Paleo Salad Recipes for Optimal Health & Nutrition

96. Shredded Chicken with Stir Fried Alkaline Vegetables

Servings: 2-3

Preparation time: 20 minutes

There's nothing more delicious and nutritious than chicken. Combine it with alkaline vegetables and you get the most energy filled lunch.

Ingredients:

- 1 tablespoon olive oil
- 1 bowl of chopped Zucchini
- 1 bowl shredded cabbage
- 1 bowl of yellow, red and green bell peppers
- Two onions roughly sliced
- 3-4 Garlic cloves
- 1 bowl of carrots
- 1 tablespoon almonds
- 1 cup (250gr) shredded chicken (you can use some leftovers)
- Salt to taste

Preparation

1. Chop zucchini, bell peppers, carrots and set them aside. Cut thin slices of garlic cloves.
2. Take a sauce pan and put one tablespoon of olive oil in it. Put it on slow heat and then add sliced garlic to it. 3.
3. When the garlic turns light brown, add onions and sauté for a while. Later add all the sliced vegetables and fry them for about 5 minutes on medium heat.
4. Now add the chicken sprinkle some salt as per your taste and cover it with a lid.
5. Stir-fry for about 10 minutes, the cool down and serve.

Serving

Serve in a colored plate and decorate it with a slice of pineapple on the side. To add some more crunch to it, you can use chopped parsley or spinach, deep fry it and sprinkle it on top of this dish. Alternatively you can always add some fresh greens.

97. Easy Salad Wrap

Servings: 2-3

Preparation time: 15 minutes

Chicken, as we all know contains substantial amount of proteins. Be sure to use organic, free range chicken for maximum benefits.

Ingredients

- 4-5 iceberg or Romanian lettuce leaves
- 2-3 avocados
- 2 ripe tomatoes
- 1 chopped onion + 1 for garnishing
- 1 cup shredded chicken
- Some parsley
- Some salt to taste
- 1 pinch of pepper powder
- 1 teaspoon lime juice
- 2 sheets of gluten-free paleo-friendly tortillas

Preparation

1. The first step is to mash the ripe avocadoes properly. Slice the tomatoes, onion, parsley and Romanian lettuce.
2. Now put these ingredients in a large bowl and add pieces of chicken to it. Squeeze some lime juice into it. Add salt, some pepper powder and toss it well.

3. Take tortilla sheets and place them on a tray. Now carefully fill them with the salad mixture and roll them. You can secure the roll with a toothpick.

Serving

Take a couple of lettuce leaves and place them on a large white dish, one on top of the other. Now place the tortillas on top of them and serve. You can insert a couple of olives or cherry tomatoes on the tip of the toothpick to make it look more appealing. You can serve this wrap with a coconut yogurt and mint dip.

98 Paleo Salmon Salad

Salmon is an excellent, lean source of protein as well as healthy omega acids.

It is low in sodium which makes it a nice addition to the alkaline diet. My Paleo style husband loves it too. This salad is really quick to prepare, raw and high in nutrients. A recommend for Alkaline Paleo fans as well.

Servings: 4

Preparation time: max 20 minutes

Ingredients:

- A few strips of smoked salmon, cut into smaller pieces
- Half cup of almonds
- 2 carrots, peeled (unless organic) and sliced
- 1 cucumber, peeled and sliced
- 1 onion, minced
- 2 cups of baby spinach
- 4 big tomatoes, sliced
- 2 garlic cloves, minced
- 2 big peppers, chopped
- Optional: ¼ of iceberg lettuce
- Juice of 1 lemon and olive oil

- Himalaya salt and rosemary herb

Preparation:

1. Wash all the ingredients, peel and chop.
2. Mix in a big bowl.
3. Sprinkle over some olive oil and lemon juice.
4. Add Himalaya salt to taste.
5. Enjoy, we do!

99. *Mediterranean Omega Salad with Tuna*

Another quick recipe inspired by traditional Southern European Diet.

Servings: 4

Preparation time: max 10 minutes

Ingredients:

- Half iceberg lettuce, washed, dried and chopped
- 1 cup of baby spinach, washed, dried and chopped
- 1 big avocado, washed, peeled, pitted and chopped
- 2 cans of tuna
- 2 tomatoes, washed and sliced
- 2 carrots, washed, peeled (unless organic) and sliced
- 2 cucumbers, washed, peeled and sliced
- 1 big onion, minced
- 2 garlic cloves, peeled and minced
- Olive oil
- Juice of 2 lemons
- Optional: 2 tablespoons of soy lecithin granules (equals to better memory and concentration- great for both kids and adults)

Instructions:

1. Simply mix all the veggies and pasta in a big bowl.
2. Sprinkle over some olive oil and lemon juice.

3. Add salt to taste. Enjoy!

100. Easy Veggie Salad

Servings: 2

Preparation time: max 15 minutes

Ingredients:

- 2 big apples, peeled, pitted and chopped
- 1 avocado, peeled, pitted and chopped
- 2 tomatoes, slices
- 2 carrots, peeled and sliced
- 1 big pepper (green, red or orange), sliced
- Juice of 1 lemon
- Olive oil
- Himalaya Salt
- 1 cup of green olives, pitted
- A few raisins

Instructions:

1. Mix all the ingredients in a bowl.
2. Add olive oil, lemon juice and Himalaya salt.
3. Don't forget about olives and raisins! An excellent combination.

101. Color Stir Fry

Servings: 4

Preparation time: max 20 minutes

Ingredients:

- A few slices of salmon, bacon or other protein of your choice
- 1 big onion, peeled and minced
- 2 garlic cloves, peeled and minced
- Coconut oil
- A few tablespoons of coconut milk
- A few big peppers (green, red and yellow), I usually go for 6 big peppers of mixed colors
- 2 zucchini
- Himalayan Salt

Preparation:

1. In a saucepan, heat up a few tablespoons of coconut oil.
2. Add garlic and onions and stir for a few minutes.
3. Add salmon (or bacon). Fry for a few minutes.
4. Add salt and a bit of coconut milk. Lower the heat.
5. Add chopped veggies and stir-fry until soft (low heat, 15 minutes).
6. Serve with a few lime or lemon slices.
7. Enjoy!

102. Carrots Aperitif

This is a fantastic alkaline aperitif...

Servings: 2

Preparation time: max 10 minutes

Ingredients:

- 3, 4 carrots, (cut in smaller sticks)
- 1 cucumber
- 1 avocado
- 2 tomatoes
- 2 tablespoons of coconut oil
- Himalayan salt

Preparation:

1. Blend avocado + tomatoes + cucumber.
2. Add some coconut oil and mix.
3. Add salt and pepper to taste.
4. Serve with carrot sticks. Cucumber sticks or radishes are also great.
5. Enjoy, we love this quick recipe when awaiting our main dish!

OPTIONAL- you can use it as raw alkaline salad dressing for other salads of your choice

Finally,

We hope you enjoyed the recipes!

If you have a second, please leave us an honest review, it would be really much appreciated.

Just let us know your favorite recipe(s).

We would love to hear from you!

CONCLUSION

Thanks again for taking interest in my book.

Now take your time to master the skill of healthy meal preparation. Invest in your health- the best asset you can possibly create.

Remember to subscribe to our free Alkaline Paleo newsletter and get a free instant access to Alkaline Paleo Superfoods!

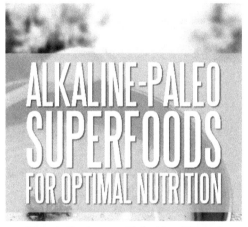

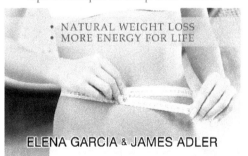

Visit: www.YourWellnessBooks.com/newsletter

And become a successful reader at no cost!

For more books and eBooks, visit:

www.YourWellnessBooks.com

In case you have questions, suggestions or doubts please e-mail me at: info@yourwellnessbooks.com

Thanks again for purchasing my book. I wish you lots of success with your health goals!

Elena Garcia

9 781913 517618